Runner's World

VITAMIN BOOK

Runner's World

VITAMIN BOOK

by Virginia DeMoss

Runner's World Books

Library of Congress Cataloging in Publication Data

DeMoss, Virginia, 1948-
   Runner's world vitamin book.
  (Instructional book/Runner's World Books;9)

  1.Vitamins I.Runner's world II. Title
QP771.D45   641.1'8   82-385
ISBN: 0-89037-146-6   AACR2

©1982 by
Virginia DeMoss

Contents

Acknowledgments vi
Introduction vii
PART ONE
OUR NEED FOR VITAMINS .1
  1. Recommended Daily Allowances (RDA) 3
  2. How Vitamins Are Measured 13
PART TWO
VITAMINS A THROUGH K .17
  3. How Vitamins Are Made 19
  4. Vitamin A 33
  5. Thiamin (B1) 41
  6. Riboflavin (B2) 47
  7. Niacin (B3) 51
  8. Vitamin B6 (Pyridoxine) 59
  9. Folacin 65
10. Vitamin B12 (Cobalamin) 71
11. Biotin 77
12. Pantothenic Acid 81
13. Vitamin C (Ascorbic Acid) 85
14. Vitamin D 97
15. Vitamin E (Tocopherol) 105
16. Vitamin K 113
PART THREE
MINERALS AND NON-VITAMINS 117
17. Non-Vitamins 119
18. Minerals 129
PART FOUR
VITAMINS IN FOOD 137
19. Are You Coming Up Short? 139
20. Getting Your Vitamins From Food 147
PART FIVE
LABELS, ALCOHOL AND PICKING PILLS 159
21. Reading Nutrition Labels 161
22. Drugs, Alcohol and Tobacco vs. Vitamins 171
23. Picking a Pill 177
24. Natural Vitamins vs. Synthetic 185
Bibliography 195
Recommended Reading 200
About the Author 201

Acknowledgments

First, the emotional thank-yous: To my parents, Virginia De-Moss and Ray DeMoss, who between them managed to give me an ability to write, a desire to get things done and a great regard for the truth. To my sister Wrayanne for the beautiful working space, the two entertaining cats that go with it, and much more. To my sister Krista and the rest of my family for their sense of humor. To my friend Cynthia Galles for reading this and other manuscripts and having the intelligence and courage to make constructive criticism. To my friend Irma Hutton for providing the constant encouragement that helps get a project like this completed. To all my friends who continue to call and visit a lunatic who has become hopelessly obsessed with vitamins.

Now, the professional thank-yous: To Dr. Carol Grimes, professor of chemistry and nutrition at Goldenwest College in Westminster, California, for reviewing this manuscript and for always generously providing her sensible views of nutrition, against which I can gauge everything else I read and hear. And to all the companies, agencies, organizations and people—particularly Patricia Hausman at the Center For Science in the Public Interest and Robert J. Avery, Jr. of the National Cancer Institute—who responded so quickly and generously to my requests for information.

Photos in Chapter 3 of the vitamin tablet-making process are by Julian Baum.

We thank William T. Thompson Company for permission to photograph their facility and Semper/Moser Associates for making the arrangements.

Introduction

Of the more than forty nutrients known to be necessary to sustain human life, none has been so misunderstood, so misrepresented, or so controversial as the group known as vitamins. These minute substances got off on the wrong foot right from the start when they were christened *vitamines* in 1912 by the Polish scientist Casimir Funk because he believed they were essential to *vita* ("life") and contained amino acids. Old Casimir was only half right: vitamins are, indeed, essential for human life. However, while vitamin B1 or thiamin—with whose discovery Funk is credited—is indeed an amine (an organic compound containing nitrogen), it was later learned that not all vitamins are amines. Actually, English biochemist Frederick G. Hopkins probably came closer to the ideal name for vitamins six years earlier than Funk when he called them "accessory factors" and, based on deprivation studies with mice, described them as essential substances contained in foods.

When it comes to vitamins, there is almost nothing that is universally agreed upon, including a precise definition or even the total number of existing vitamins. It is generally held that vitamins are organic compounds that are necessary in the diet in minute amounts to perform specific metabolic functions. Unlike the macronutrients—protein, carbohydrates and fats—which are required by the body in large amounts and provide energy, vitamins are micronutrients required in trace amounts. While they do not themselves produce energy, many of them function in the conversion of food to energy.

Such a non-exclusive definition has given rise to some controversy over what substances can actually be classified as vitamins. Currently there are only thirteen recognized vitamin substances—A, B1 (thiamin), B2 (riboflavin), niacin, B6 (pyridoxine), folacin, B12, biotin, pantothenic acid, C (ascorbic acid), D, E and K— though vitamin status has been claimed for substances lettered all the way up to U. Some of these letter designations (i.e., B17 for laetrile) have simply been applied at the whim of the substance's promoters. Others were applied to substances actually thought to be new vitamins at the time of their discovery. Later, some of these failed to meet the criteria for being called a vitamin, while others were found to be vitamins already discovered. In the case of the B-complex, after its inital discovery it was learned that B was not a single compound but a number of separate ones, so number designations were applied to distinguish one from another. Today, to avoid the confusion of letters and numbers, vitamins are often referred to by their chemical names.

Vitamins are, appropriately, sometimes termed "regulatory nutrients" for their function of choreographing the body's chemical reactions. Although, as health writer Phyllis Lehmann has pointed out, "They do not directly provide energy or build any part of the body, they are required for, among other things, new cell growth, proper digestion, nerve function, and conversion of food into energy." Many vitamins help carry out chemical reactions in the body by acting as coenzymes.

Lack of a particular vitamin will produce a specific deficiency disease. In 1747, physician James Lind believed that oranges and lemons were the cure for scurvy, the disease characterized by weakness, anemia, spongy gums and bleeding from the mucous membranes, that was rapidly depleting the British Navy. He was right, although the responsible agent, vitamin C, was not isolated until 1932 and called ascorbic (meaning "without scurvy") acid. Since Lind's day a number of the world's other dread diseases have been cured by vitamin substances isolated from food. Among them are rickets (softening and bending of the bones), beriberi (weakness, paralysis, anemia and wasting away), pellagra (gastrointestinal disturbances, skin eruptions, nervous disorders), and pernicious anemia. The substances that get the credit are, respectively, vitamin D, thiamin, niacin and B12.

Vitamins are of two types: water-soluble (B-complex and C), found only in the portion of foods soluble in water, and fat-soluble (A,D,E,K). Though the body can use the same vitamins again and again, they are eventually broken down, changed, or, in the case of the water-solubles, excreted in the urine. Fat-soluble vitamins are accumulated in the liver and other organs and fatty tissues of the body and are not as rapidly cleared out of the system. Most vitamins, as their definition indicates, come to us in the food we eat, but some are produced, at least in part, within the body. Synthesis of some vitamins is performed by bacterial action in the intestines. It is not often clear just how much usable vitamin is provided in this way. In addition, vitamin D is produced by sunlight reacting with the cells under the skin's surface, and the amino acid tryptophan can be converted to niacin. Additionally, plant foods contain not vitamin A, but carotene, the precursor from which A is manufactured in the body.

Many of the vitamins are not single compounds, but a group of several with similar chemical structure and activity. Vitamin E, for example, is the generic name given to a number of tocopherols and tocotrienols, both naturally occurring and synthetic. In this case not all of the forms are equally active; the other forms are estimated to have anywhere from 1 to 50 percent of the strength of alpha-tocopherol, the most common and biologically active of the E substances. In the case of some vitamins, the various forms are converted to a single active form in the body.

As vitamins were discovered—most often through their role in dramatically curing a deficiency disease—there began the long, difficult process of determining their necessary amounts for human health and the extent to which they occurred in foods. In 1943 the Food and Nutrition Board of the National Academy of Sciences, National Research Council, brought some order and precision to the activity by publishing the first Recommended Dietary Allowances, estimated optimum intakes of vitamins, minerals and other nutrients, based on the Board's review of all existing evidence. The RDAs, which have their equivalents in other countries, are updated approximately every five years, and, despite criticism generated mainly by megavitamin proponents, are still the most accurate estimates we have of the average individual's nutrient needs. It is very important to remember when using the RDAs as a dietary guide that their numbers do not represent minimum requirements for nutrients, but include a generous margin of safety so that they might represent the optimum needs of a broad cross-section of the American population.

By selecting a wide variety of foods with an eye to their nutritional content, the members of the Food and Nutrition Board and most nutritionists feel that one can be fairly certain of meeting or exceeding his or her nutritional needs as determined by the RDAs, especially since they are all optimum figures. Of course, doing so requires a modicum of effort and responsibility on the part of the consumer. He must be willing to assure that the bulk of his calorie intake comes from fresh, whole foods (believe it or not, a slightly revised version of the old "Basic Four Food Groups" is still a useful guide) rather than processed-to-death convenience foods and sugary snacks. He must also not be fooled by some "fortified" and "enriched" foods, which are often nothing more than nutritionally bereft sugar and white flour to which a tiny handful of the original nutrients have been returned. Vitamins are worthless without wholesome food on which to work. Keeping that fact in mind will also hopefully put an end to the absurd practice of downing a handful of vitamins in lieu of breakfast or another meal.

So, you might ask, if it is still possible in this day and age to meet our nutritional needs with the foods we eat, why did Americans spend $1.3 billion on vitamin supplements in 1980 (not to mention the billions spent by industry to doctor the food we eat, the food our pets eat, and even the food the animals we eat eat), and why does that figure increase by 10 percent annually? A good question. Vitamins—on the basis of both outrageous claims and some promising research—have come to be regarded by some—and often the better educated among us—as substances of almost miraculous powers. Just ask any of sixty million Americans who will tell you that vitamins will give you more pep, knock out a cold, improve your sex life, or at least your athletic performance, and cure cancer.

While there are still areas where deficiency diseases persist, the average middle-class American is seldom plagued by scurvy or beriberi. That is not to say, however, that there may not be "borderline" or "subclinical" deficiencies among the population at large, though these are difficult to assess. If they do exist, it is, again, probably due to our rather lazy attitudes toward food. In addition, there are some specialized groups that researchers are coming to regard as prime targets of deficiencies.

The elderly is one group that generally must try to get the same number of nutrients with less money, less effort, and usually less appetite. For them, supplementation is often recommended. A common deficiency among many women and children is not of a vitamin, but the mineral iron. For some, getting enough iron in the diet, even with very careful food selection, is extremely difficult. Pregnant, lactating and menstruating women may have other increased needs, as well, particularly for calcium, folacin and some of the other B vitamins, but should check with their doctors regarding supplementation.

As medical writer Arielle Emmett points out, "Women on oral contraceptives number about ten million in this country, and are highly susceptible to reduced (but not always deficient) levels of C, thiamin, riboflavin, cyanocobalamin, pyridoxine, and folic acid." As some researchers feel supplements are essential for these women, others say that while there may be reduced levels of certain vitamins, there is no proof of serious vitamin deficiency. It's a good idea to check with the doctor who fills your prescription for the Pill for advice regarding supplementation.

Vegans (strict vegetarians who consume no eggs or dairy products) could possibly become deficient in certain nutrients (B12 is the major problem), and there are, of course, those rare few who are suffering disorders that prevent them from utilizing vitamins properly. Those who are chronically ill or under stress may have increased vitamin needs, as well.

There are certain other groups that vitamin enthusiasts often point to as having increased vitamin needs. Cigarette smoking, for example, is thought to rapidly deplete vitamin C. Alcohol, too, can have an effect on the absorption of vitamins, and very heavy drinkers—who often substitute liquor for food—are prone to malnutrition. Others who can run into trouble are drug users (prescription, over-the-counter and recreational), those who get a high percentage of their calories from sweets or other "empty" foods, and those whose sedentary lifestyles have forced them to cut down on calories—and thus nutrients—in order to keep their weight down. Some vitamin companies and authors have recommended vitamin supplementation of various types for all of the above-mentioned groups, though other sources claim that levels, even if lowered, are still easily within the safe range.

Ah, the American Dream. Why stop smoking, eat right or exercise when you can indulge in unhealthy or excessive habits and take a magic pill to make you better? In many cases, the biggest deficiency Americans have is not one of vitamins, but willpower, and it's the rare manufacturer who isn't willing to exploit that fact. This is not meant to be self-righteous or to imply that alcoholism, for instance, constitutes a lack of willpower and not a serious illness, or that other habits are easy to break; it means simply that there is no easy substitute—vitamins included—for proper care of the body.

There is cause to be concerned about the nutritional value of many of the foods we consume today (if we succumb to convenience and fast foods), but our markets are still well-stocked with nutritious whole foods, and these are the best way to get the vitamins *and* dozens of other nutrients we need. Vitamins are needed by the body in very minute quantities—even deficiency diseases are corrected by relatively small doses. If you are not suffering from a deficiency disease but are still worried about a "borderline" deficiency of vitamins or minerals in your diet, due to ingestion of a certain number of processed foods, concern over the nutritional content of fruits and vegetables that may have sat on the grocer's shelf too long, the unavailability of fresh produce, or any of a number of other reasons, a simple multiple vitamin/mineral tablet that contains no more than the RDA for each substance should be all the insurance you need. Once a deficiency is made up—if it did indeed exist—any excess vitamins you consume provide no further *nutritional* action; they are either stored in the tissues (the implications of which will be discussed), or flushed out of the body, creating, as a common joke goes, very expensive urine.

In recent years nearly all of us have become familiar with the term "megavitamin therapy," which consists of the administration of vitamins in "megadoses" that are sometimes ten, twenty or even a hundred or thousand times above recommended levels. The growing popularity of megadosing is based on a number of factors: some promising case studies and scientific evidence; some as yet unproven or totally unfounded claims by certain vitamin manufacturers, health food faddists and other "experts;" the typically American notion that if a little of something is good, a whole lot must be better; the widely held belief that because they are "natural" substances, vitamins can't be harmful in any quantity, and, last but not least, Linus Pauling and his optimistic claims for vitamin C.

There is an important distinction between a vitamin's "vitamin" or "nutritional" effect and its "pharmacological" or "drug" effect. Respected nutritionist Dr. Jean Mayer, formerly a professor at Harvard and now president of Tufts University, explains it this way: "When you take any vitamin greatly in excess of the dosage necessary to prevent deficiency, it stops acting like a vitamin in the body. Though each vitamin has its own special role to play, and some have more than one, they all have the same general function: they act as 'coenzymes.' In the cells, these 'coenzymes' join up with proteins called 'apoenzymes' to form complete enzymes, catalysts that speed up normal, necessary metabolic reactions. However, cells can manufacture just so many 'apoenzymes.' That means that in megadoses many vitamins cannot perform their natural function, but instead act like a drug."

Some of the drug actions attributed to vitamins have already been mentioned, including curing cancer and the common cold. They also encompass the use of B1 or thiamin as a treatment for multiple sclerosis, neuritis and mental disorders, niacin for heart attacks and schizophrenia, pantothenic acid to prevent or reverse graying, A for acne, D for arthritis, and on and on. C has been touted as the cure for just about everything.

Based on the limited availability of scientific data from carefully controlled studies, such organizations as the Food and Drug Administration Advisory Panel on Vitamin and Mineral Drug Products for Over-the-Counter Human Use, the American Psychiatric Association, and the Department of Drugs of the American Medical Association, have, in the cases of specific vitamins, discounted their effectiveness against these and other diseases.

Perhaps because of vitamins' ability to dramatically cure certain diseases (scurvy, pellagra, etc.) and their function of affecting changes in the body, the role of vitamins in some as yet unconquered diseases presents some very attractive theories. While there are, of course, those who will want only to make claims of any kind to sell products, there are others who, based on individual case histories and preliminary investigations, genuinely feel that vitamins can be of use against certain diseases, and still others who are actively engaged in carefully controlled experiments to test some of the more promising theories. As things stand now, those who flatly state that vitamins are of no use at all in disease prevention and cures are probably as far off base as those who make totally unsubstantiated claims. The fact is that there is evidence to *suggest* some very attractive possibilities, but many of them are as yet unproven.

Most self-prescribed megadosing has less to do with curing illnesses than with such things as improving performance or "optimizing" health. That's the popular "if a little is good a lot must be better" theory spoken of earlier that keeps the vitamin industry healthy. Often vitamin companies or reporters for health food magazines and grocery store tabloids will push a vitamin's benefit through extrapolation. Based on what a vitamin does in standard amounts they'll support their assertions of the miraculous benefits that more of it can provide. Additionally, they often conclude that because a deficiency of a vitamin can produce a specific effect, an excess will produce the opposite desired effect. Another favorite ploy is picking up the preliminary results from an animal study and printing them as though they applied to human beings. This practice is erroneous: when it comes to nutrient reactions, species vary greatly.

No matter what the effect you desire, there is someone somewhere who has a product they will swear can achieve it....and they will be able to provide dozens of convincing reasons why. Most of them will be based on that familiar notion of "what a little will do a lot will do better." A common argument of the vitamin pushers is that just because the RDAs may be enough to prevent disease, how do we know they're optimum levels for best performance of a vitamin? Although the Food and Nutrition Board takes into account subtle changes in a vitamin's performance at different levels of intake when establishing the RDAs, there probably are many things we have yet to learn. But then it must be remembered that megavitamin proponents do not have access to some secret or special knowledge; they have no better idea than anyone else what the ideal levels are. Their recommendations of 10 grams of this to prevent colds, 25,000 milligrams of that for better endurance and 5000 IU of something else for joint lubrication are simply a matter of guesswork.

Especially susceptible to such claims are athletes who are always trying to maximize performance. Thus, there is a raft of supplement products aimed at athletes in general and runners in particular. It's a good idea to be especially wary of those who tell you that RDAs are compiled by inaccurate guesswork and hocus-pocus based on non-existent "typical Americans," and then say in the same breath that they know exactly what vitamin formulation the "typical runner" needs. Actually, most athletes, because of increased calorie intakes and a generally higher regard for good nutrition, are one of the *least* likely groups to need supplementation. (Those who wish to pursue this subject further are referred to the following articles: "Olympic Athletes View Vitamins and Victory," by Elington Darden and "Nutrition and Athletics," by Olaf Mickelsen; both are collected in *The Nutrition Crisis*, edited by Theodore P. Labuza (St. Paul: West Publishing Co., 1975), and

"Nutrition and Athletic Performance," by the Dairy Council, contained in *Contemporary Nutrition Controversies,* edited by Labuza and A. Elizabeth Sloan (St. Paul: West Publishing Co., 1979).

When you come across a supplement developed specifically for the runner, forget the claims a minute and read the label. Maybe that substance touted to "repair cartilage and aid in detoxification" is nothing more than high-potency vitamin C, or the one that combats stress is simply a high-dosage vitamin/mineral capsule. It's a good bet, though, that you will pay several times more for those common supplements in a bottle designed for runners only than you will to get them in a bottle geared for the population at large.

In the long run, like most things, the decision of whether to dose yourself with large quantities of vitamins is yours. The best advice anyone can give you is to read the claims, consider their source, and carefully evaluate the evidence....if any is given. Only claims backed up by carefully controlled experiments (on human beings) should be taken seriously, and often that information is difficult for the lay public to get and to evaluate.

One variable that mars many experiments is the very real "placebo effect." Often, being told they are being administered a substance to improve their health or performance (even if it is just a sugar pill), will provide subjects with the needed psychological boost. In *Vitamins: Their Use and Abuse,* Joseph V. Levy and Paul Bach-y-Rita maintain that "a rational evaluation of vitamins must lead to the conclusion that many of the apparently miraculous effects claimed for vitamins are a result of the power of suggestion, and that any other substance that could inspire as much faith would have similar effects."

One of the vitamin purveyor's best arguments has been that even if large quantities of vitamins can't help you, they can't hurt you, so it's better to play it safe. Not only is that an expensive proposition, but mounting evidence suggests that just the opposite may be true, that "playing it safe" might be better accomplished by letting the diet supply vitamins and minerals.

First of all, we know that many vitamins work by interaction with one another. Ingestion of high doses of one can affect levels of others, throwing off the body's delicate balance. That's yet another good reason to try to get what we need from our food.

We know also that the levels of fat-soluble vitamins our bodies can't use are stored in the tissues. It has been proven that mega-dosing on A, D and K can be toxic. Yet it is a commonly held misconception that these are the only vitamins that are potentially harmful. The water-soluble vitamins, in particular, are regarded as safe because the body is thought to simply flush out what it doesn't use. But there is increasing evidence that large doses of C and some of the Bs can also cause problems while just passing through. Some difficulties possibly related to excessive doses of vitamin C, for example, are kidney stones and severe diarrhea. Minerals, too, can cause serious problems in excess, as can some of the non-vitamin substances. Many supplements come packed with high doses of these so-called vitamins that we know very little about. Since we really don't have a clear picture of what the body does with such substances—or whether we need some of them at all—it seems rather risky to ingest large supplemental amounts of them.

Although overdosing on vitamins is not a good idea for anyone, it is especially to be avoided by pregnant or lactating women. (Don't confuse overdosing with taking necessary supplements your physician may suggest). Such women are putting another system besides their own at risk and taking the very real risk of doing harm to the child or producing a child with a life-long vitamin dependency.

While some vitamin substances *appear* to be relatively safe in megadoses over the short haul, we really won't know what their prolonged use will do until, as chemist and nutritionist Dr. Carol Grimes points out, "there have been a lot of people who have been taking large amounts for a very long time. It's not clear whether there are going to be any long-term serious effects. We just simply have to wait and see." The information on the following pages can serve as a guide to the *known* risks and advantages of vitamin use, but only time will tell whether we, the most health-conscious gen-eration in history, are helping or harming ourselves and our off-spring with our current vitamin obsession.

PART ONE
OUR NEED FOR VITAMINS

NUTRITION INFORMATION

SERVING SIZE: 1 OZ. (28.4 g, ABOUT ¾ CUP) CEREAL ALONE OR WITH ½ CUP VITAMIN D FORTIFIED WHOLE MILK.

SERVINGS PER PACKAGE: 12

	FLAKES OF WHOLE WHEAT	
	CEREAL	WITH MILK
CALORIES	110	180
PROTEIN	3 g	7 g
CARBOHYDRATE	24 g	30 g
FAT	0 g	4 g
SODIUM	195 mg	255 mg
	(680 mg per 100 g)	(170 mg per 100 g)

PERCENTAGE OF U.S. RECOMMENDED DAILY ALLOWANCES (U.S. RDA)

	FLAKES OF WHOLE WHEAT	
	CEREAL	WITH MILK
PROTEIN	4	15
VITAMIN A	25	30
VITAMIN C	25	25
THIAMIN	25	30
RIBOFLAVIN	25	35
NIACIN	25	25
CALCIUM	*	15
IRON	4	4
VITAMIN D	10	25
VITAMIN E	25	25
VITAMIN B₆	25	30
FOLIC ACID	25	25
VITAMIN B₁₂	25	30
PHOSPHORUS	10	20
MAGNESIUM	6	10
ZINC	25	30
COPPER	8	8

*CONTAINS LESS THAN 2% OF THE U.S. RDA OF THIS NUTRIENT.

1

Recommended Daily
Allowances (RDA)

While vitamin proponents preach the glories of megadoses, most nutritionists continue to thump their own bible: the RDAs. It has long been known that adequate amounts of certain nutrients can promote general health and prevent a number of specific deficiency diseases (i.e., scurvy, beriberi, rickets, pellagra, anemias, etc.). But what those adequate amounts are is a question that has plagued nutritionists, doctors and public health officials for decades. The quest for the optimal diet for the American public seemed a particularly important goal during World War II; thus, in 1943, the Food and Nutrition Board of the National Academy of Sciences—National Research Council, published the first Recommended Dietary Allowances (RDAs) as a "guide for planning and procuring food supplies for national defense."

The RDAs have been revised approximately every five years since their initial publication and their role has been greatly expanded. Today their usefulness extends to such activities as "interpreting food consumption records of groups and evaluating the adequacy of food supplies in meeting nutritional needs, planning and procuring food supplies for groups and establishing guides for public food assistance programs, development of new food products by industry, establishing guidelines for nutritional labeling of foods, and developing nutrition education programs."

The Ninth Edition (1980) of the RDAs includes estimated optimum intakes of ten vitamins and six minerals for seventeen different groups of people (i.e., infants in two age groups, children in three age groups, males and females in five age groups each, and pregnant and lactating women). In the Ninth Edition, the RDAs also list "Estimated Safe and Adequate Daily Dietary Intakes of

3

Selected Vitamins and Minerals." These nutrients, which include biotin, pantothenic acid and vitamin K, are listed in a separate table because there is less scientific data on which to base their suggested intakes. Most of these are listed as ranges of safe intake; based on available evidence, intakes that fall within these ranges are probably neither inadequate nor excessive. Because less is known about them, levels for nutrients in this table are established for only seven age groups.

The RDAs are the product of a review of all pertinent scientific data, epidemiological evidence (examining deficient populations and quantities of nutrients required to correct deficiencies), and expensive and time-consuming testing that includes evaluations of the nutrient intake and excretion of normal, healthy people, biochemical measurements of body levels of nutrients, controlled experiments with induced deficiencies (when such studies present no risk to the subjects involved), and, occasionally, extrapolation from animal studies.

One of the most important points to remember about the RDAs is that they are not hard-and-fast rules that every individual must adhere to, nor are they minimum dietary requirements. As the introduction to the RDA Tables advises, "RDA are recommendations for the average daily amounts of nutrients that *population groups* should consume over a period of time. RDA should not be confused with requirements for a specific individual. Differences in the nutrient requirements of individuals are ordinarily unknown. Therefore, RDA (except for energy) are estimated to exceed the requirements of most individuals and thereby to ensure that the needs of nearly all in the population are met. Intakes below the recommended allowance for a nutrient are not necessarily inadequate, but the risk of having an inadequate intake increases to the extent that intake is less than the level recommended as safe."

Here are some other important things to remember about the RDAs:

● RDAs meet the needs of most healthy individuals and provide a generous margin of safety. They do not, however, take into account increased nutrient needs associated with such problems as absorptive disorders, chronic disease, premature birth, special medications, etc. Also, nutrient needs may vary with such things as climate and physical activity. Because the RDAs are not hard-and-fast rules and provide a generous margin of safety, they should be good guidelines under most circumstances. However, special situations may also carry with them an automatic adjustment in nutrient intake. For the athlete, for example, increased expenditure of energy leads to increased food intake and, therefore, increased nutrients.

● RDAs have not been set for all of the nutrients known to be necessary for the health of humans. It is intended, therefore, that the RDAs be met by a varied diet to assure that other nutrient needs are met, as well.

● The RDAs take into account the absorption efficiency of nutrients, as well as the rate at which precursor forms are converted to active vitamins. The figures adequately provide for the difference between what is consumed and what is actually available for use. Since, for example, only a part of dietary iron is absorbed and much of it is excreted, the RDA for iron is set high enough to assure that we get enough usable mineral. Thus, when you hear that only a fraction of a nutrient is absorbed or made available for use, you don't have to increase your intake to be sure you get the recommended amount. That has already been done for you.

● RDAs for some nutrients exceed the presumed requirement by more than others. According to the statement prepared by the Committee, "On the whole, those who accept responsibility for estimating allowances tend to select the higher of alternate levels when there is little evidence that small surpluses of nutrients are detrimental."

● Although the RDAs are listed as daily allowances, due to storage of most vitamins and various protective mechanisms of the body, it is not necessary to get all nutrients in the prescribed quantities every day. The Food and Nutrition Board, in fact, suggests averaging nutrient intakes over a five-to eight-day period.

● Most, but not all, nutrients are tolerated well in amounts that exceed the allowances by as much as two to three times.

While it is certainly true that no two individuals have identical needs, it is generally agreed upon among responsible nutritionists that, based on the evidence currently available, using the RDAs as *guidelines* (not absolute dictates), is a pretty effective way to assure optimum nutrition.

RECOMMENDED DIETARY ALLOWANCES (RDAs)
REVISED 1980

"Designed for the maintenance of good nutrition of practically all healthy people in the U.S.A."

Fat-Soluble Vitamins

	Age (years)	Vitamin A (mcg RE)*	Vitamin D (ug)	Vitamin E (mg ∝TE)**
Infants	0.0-0.5	420	10	3
	0.5-1.0	400	10	4
Children	1-3	400	10	5
	4-6	500	10	6
	7-10	700	10	7
Males	11-14	1000	10	8
	15-18	1000	10	10
	19-22	1000	7.5	10
	23-50	1000	5	10
	51+	1000	5	10
Females	11-14	800	10	8
	15-18	800	10	8
	19-22	800	7.5	8
	23-50	800	5	8
	51+	800	5	8
Pregnant		+200	+5	+2
Lactating		+400	+5	+3

*Retinol Equivalents
**Alpha-tocopherol Equivalents

(cont. next page)

(cont. from previous page)

RECOMMENDED DIETARY ALLOWANCES (RDAs)
REVISED 1980

Water-Soluble Vitamins

	Age (years)	Vitamin C (mg)	Thiamin (mg)	Riboflavin (mg)	Niacin (mg NE)***
Infants	0.0-0.5	35	0.3	0.4	6
	0.5-1.0	35	0.5	0.6	8
Children	1-3	45	0.7	0.8	9
	4-6	45	0.9	1.0	11
	7-10	45	1.2	1.4	16
Males	11-14	50	1.4	1.6	18
	15-18	60	1.4	1.7	18
	19-22	60	1.5	1.7	19
	23-50	60	1.4	1.6	18
	51+	60	1.2	1.4	16
Females	11-14	50	1.1	1.3	15
	15-18	60	1.1	1.3	14
	19-22	60	1.1	1.3	14
	23-50	60	1.0	1.2	13
	51+	60	1.0	1.2	13
Pregnant		+20	+0.4	+0.3	+2
Lactating		+40	+0.5	+0.5	+5

***Niacin Equivalents

(cont next page)

RECOMMENDED DIETARY ALLOWANCES (RDAs)
REVISED 1980

	Age (years)	Water-Soluble Vitamins (cont.)			Minerals
		Vita-min B-6 (mg)	Fola-cin (mcg)	Vitamin B-12 (mcg)	Cal-cium (mg)
Infants	0.0-0.5	0.3	30	0.5	360
	0.5-1.0	0.6	45	1.5	540
Children	1-3	0.9	100	2.0	800
	4-6	1.3	200	2.5	800
	7-10	1.6	300	3.0	800
Males	11-14	1.8	400	3.0	1200
	15-18	2.0	400	3.0	1200
	19-22	2.2	400	3.0	800
	23-50	2.2	400	3.0	800
	51+	2.2	400	3.0	800
Females	11-14	1.8	400	3.0	1200
	15-18	2.0	400	3.0	1200
	19-22	2.0	400	3.0	800
	23-50	2.0	400	3.0	800
	51+	2.0	400	3.0	800
Pregnant		+0.6	+400	+1.0	+400
Lactating		+0.5	+100	+1.0	+400

(cont. next page)

(cont. from previous page)

RECOMMENDED DIETARY ALLOWANCES (RDAs)
REVISED 1980

Minerals (cont.)

	Phos-phorus (mg)	Mag-nesium (mg)	Iron (mg)	Zinc (mg)	Iodine (mcg)
Infants	240	50	10	3	40
	360	70	15	5	50
Children	800	150	15	10	70
	800	200	10	10	90
	800	250	10	10	120
Males	1200	350	18	15	150
	1200	400	18	15	150
	800	350	10	15	150
	800	350	10	15	150
	800	350	10	15	150
Females	1200	300	18	15	150
	1200	300	18	15	150
	800	300	18	15	150
	800	300	18	15	150
	800	300	10	15	150
Pregnant	+400	+150	*h* ****	+5	+25
Lactating	+400	+150	*h*	+10	+50

**** The increased requirement during pregnancy cannot be met by the iron content of habitual American diets nor by the existing iron stores of many women; therefore the use of 30-60 mg of supplemental iron is recommended. Iron needs during lactation are not substantially different from those of nonpregnant women, but continued supplementation of the mother for 2-3 months after parturition is advisable in order to replenish stores depleted by pregnancy.

Source: Food and Nutrition Board, National Academy of Sciences National Research Council

ESTIMATED SAFE AND ADEQUATE DAILY DIETARY INTAKES OF SELECTED VITAMINS AND MINERALS, 1980

Vitamins

	Age (years)	Vitamin K (mcg)	Biotin (mcg)	Pantothenic Acid (mg)
Infants	0-0.5	12	35	2
	0.5-1	10-20	50	3
Children	1-3	15-30	65	3
and	4-6	20-40	85	3-4
Adolescents	7-10	30-60	120	4-5
	11+	50-100	100-200	4-7
Adults		70-140	100-200	4-7

Trace Elements *

	Age (years)	Copper (mg)	Manganese (mg)	Fluoride (mg)	Chromium (mg)	Selenium (mg)	Molybdenum (mg)
Infants	0-0.5	0.5-0.7	0.5-0.7	0.1-0.5	0.01-0.04	0.01-0.04	0.03-0.06
	0.5-1	0.7-1.0	0.7-1.0	0.2-1.0	0.02-0.06	0.02-0.06	0.04-0.08
Children	1-3	1.0-1.5	1.0-1.5	0.5-1.5	0.02-0.08	0.02-0.08	0.05-0.1
and	4-6	1.5-2.0	1.5-2.0	1.0-2.5	0.03-0.12	0.03-0.12	0.06-0.15
Adolescents	7-10	2.0-2.5	2.0-3.0	1.5-2.5	0.05-0.2	0.05-0.2	0.10-0.3
	11+	2.0-3.0	2.5-5.0	1.5-2.5	0.05-0.2	0.05-0.2	0.15-0.5
Adults		2.0-3.0	2.5-5.0	2.5-4.0	0.05-0.2	0.05-0.2	0.15-0.5

Electrolytes

	Age (years)	Sodium (mg)	Potassium (mg)	Chloride (mg)
Infants	0-0.5	115-350	350-925	275-700
	0.5-1	250-750	425-1275	400-1200
Children	1-3	325-975	550-1650	500-1500
and	4-6	450-1350	775-2325	700-2100
Adolescents	7-10	600-1800	1000-3000	925-2775
	11+	900-2700	1525-4575	1400-4200
Adults		1100-3300	1875-5625	1700-5100

* Since the toxic levels for many trace elements may be only several times usual intakes, the upper levels for the trace elements given in this table should not be habitually exceeded.

Source: Food and Nutrition Board, National Academy of Sciences— National Research Council.

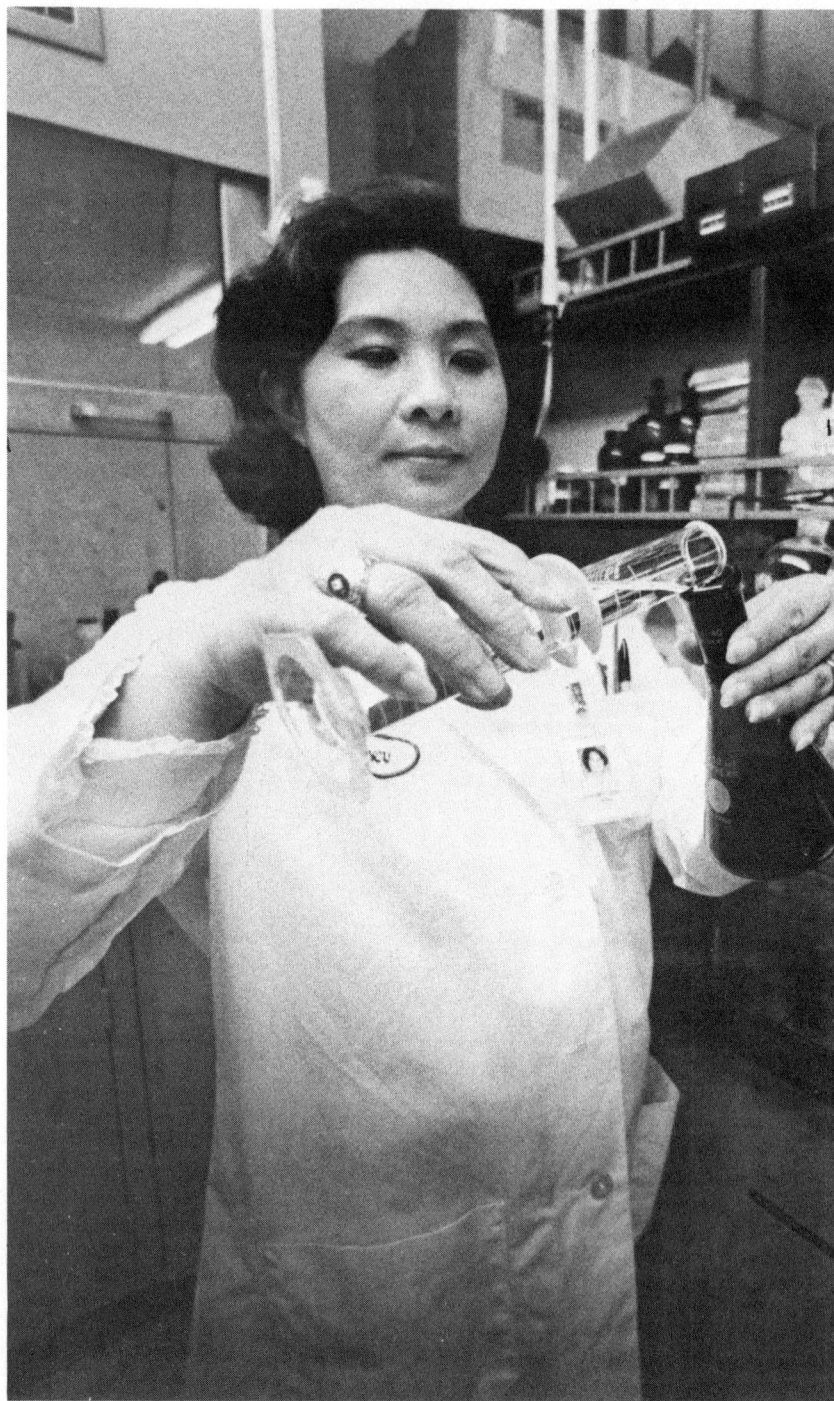

2

How Vitamins Are Measured

Selecting a vitamin supplement or planning your meals to get the Recommended Dietary Allowances of vitamins can be a little easier if you have a passing knowledge of how vitamins are measured. Until the 1980 revisions of the RDAs, the oil-soluble vitamins (A,D,E,K) were listed as IUs (International Units), according to their strength or activity, while the water-soluble vitamins (B-complex and C) were listed according to quantity, in milligrams (mg) and micrograms (mcg).

The International Unit is used to measure vitamins whose various forms differ in strength. At best, a confusing concept for the public, the IU is a standard unit that indicates the biologic activity of a vitamin or the amount needed to promote a specified growth rate in laboratory rats. It was then decided how many of those units were needed to maintain human health. Because each of the oil-soluble vitamins is different, the term IU means something different in relation to each one. For example, one IU of vitamin D measures out to 0.025 micrograms, while one IU of vitamin A is equal to 0.3 micrograms of retinol. In terms of physical size, IU means little to the public. The measurement is useful to us simply by allowing us to compare the amount of a vitamin in foods or tablets against the recommended intakes. Occasionally, oil-soluble vitamins are expressed in United States Pharmacopeia Units (USP); these do not differ significantly from IUs.

Because each type of vitamin A and provitamin A is absorbed by the body at a different rate, in 1967 the Food and Agriculture Organization/World Health Organization introduced the concept of the retinol equivalent (RE), which indicates the vitamin's activity in relation to retinol, A's active form. First, it is necessary to

13

know that vitamin A in the retinol form is totally absorbed by the body, while only one-third of the beta-carotene ingested is used and only one-half of that is converted to retinol; other carotenes have an even less efficient conversion rate. Thus, it takes six micrograms of beta-carotene to produce the effect of a single microgram of retinol. Six micrograms of beta-carotene, therefore, equal one retinol equivalent. The RE is a convenient way to sum up all the vitamin A activity from various sources.

A similar situation exists with the water-soluble vitamin niacin (B3), which not only occurs in a preformed state, but can be formed in the body from the amino acid tryptophan. To account for niacin activity, the niacin equivalent has been developed: approximately 60 mg tryptophan = 1 mg niacin = 1 niacin equivalent. (While the RDAs take into account the niacin potential of high-tryptophan foods—many listings of the nutrient content of 8.e., Agriculture Handbook No. 456—show only the amount of preformed niacin).

As noted, the other oil-soluble vitamins (D, E, and K) were also heretofore represented in the RDAs as IUs. In 1980 that changed. Vitamin E is now listed in milligrams and D and K in micrograms. The activity from all forms of these vitamins is taken into account. To put the terms "milligram" and "microgram" into perspective for you—and to illustrate just how miniscule the quantities of vitamins we need to consume are, it might be useful to know that twenty-eight grams are required to make an ounce, and that one milligram is one-thousandth of a gram, while one microgram is one-millionth of a gram! To make the point even clearer, a single ounce of vitamin B12 is enough to supply the needs of one million people.

Listing the oil-soluble vitamins in terms of REs and mg's may cause a bit of confusion for vitamin buyers, because, according to Dr. Charles Thomas of the William T. Thompson Co., a major vitamin manufacturer, they—and probably most other manufacturers—have no plans at the present time to change their labeling to match the RDA system, particularly since there are no regulations regarding vitamin labeling. As a purchaser of vitamins, your task is made somewhat easier, however, by the fact that vitamin manufacturers list the percentage of U.S. RDAs that their products contain. You can simplify the conversion for vitamin A by remembering that retinol equivalents work out to about five times less than International Units. Hence, if your supplement lists 5000 IU of vitamin A, it contains 1000 RE or the U.S. RDA. To simplify your job even more, the following tables provide translations for some common abbreviations and equivalents for various measures.

ABBREVIATIONS

RE = Retinol Equivalent
IU = International Unit
USP = United States Pharmacopeia Unit
g = gram
mg = milligram
mcg = microgram

EQUIVALENTS

454 grams = 1 pound
16 ounces = 1 pound
28 grams = 1 ounce
1000 milligrams = 1 gram
1000 micrograms = 1 milligram

VITAMIN A

1 IU = 0.3 mcg retinol, 0.6 mcg beta-carotene
1 RE = 1 mcg retinol, 6 mcg beta-carotene
1 RE = 5 IU, 3.33 IU retinol, 10 IU beta-carotene

VITAMIN B3 (NIACIN)

1 mg = 1 niacin equivalent
1 niacin equivalent = 60 mg tryptophan

VITAMIN D

1 IU = 0.025 mcg cholecalciferol
1 mcg = 40 IU

VITAMIN E

1 mg d-alpha-tocopherol = 1 alpha-tocopherol equivalent (α T.E.)
1 mg = 3 IU

PART TWO
VITAMINS A THROUGH K

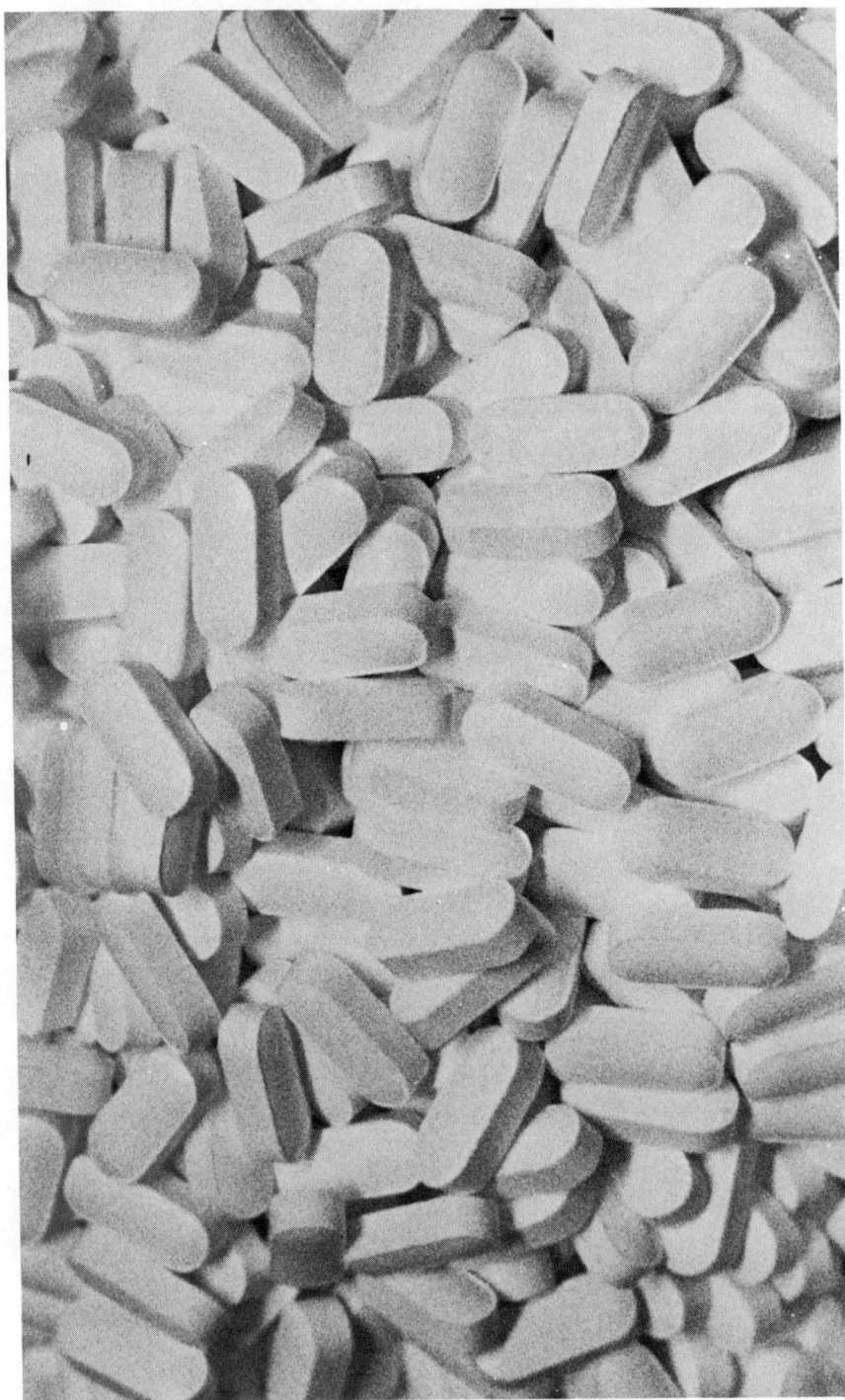

3

How Vitamins Are Made

Making vitamins into tablet-, capsule- and powder-form is a complex process, which begins in a chemistry lab. At the William T. Thompson Company's plant in Carson, California, a vast assembly line pumps out millions of vitamin tablets annually. According to Jim Hilbe, vice president of sales for William T. Thompson Company, their company is the largest supplier of vitamin products to natural food stores in the country. They supply vitamins in all fifty states and to some foreign countries.

Some 200 people work at the facility in Carson. At the chemistry lab alone, which Hilbe says is the key area in quality control, there are twenty-five chemists and technicians. To maintain cleanliness in the tablet-making process, all employees must wear uniforms, which include caps to keep out hair.

Tablet-making begins with raw material. It is mixed in a V-blender before being added to a granulating machine. After mixing and granulating, the material is spread to dry on long, flat trays. Then it is added into a tablet-compressing machine, or it might be used in capsules. Once a tablet is formed it is given a coating, which helps preserve its vitamin content. Once on the assembly line, the tablet-counter machine allows a set quantity of vitamins into a bottle; the bottle then moves down the conveyer belt, where it next receives cotton. Farther down the line the cap is automatically screwed on. Now the bottle is ready for labeling and finally, shipment.

As you might have guessed, vitamin C is the best-selling vitamin in the country. William T. Thompson Company, founded in 1935 and privately owned, issues two new products a month.

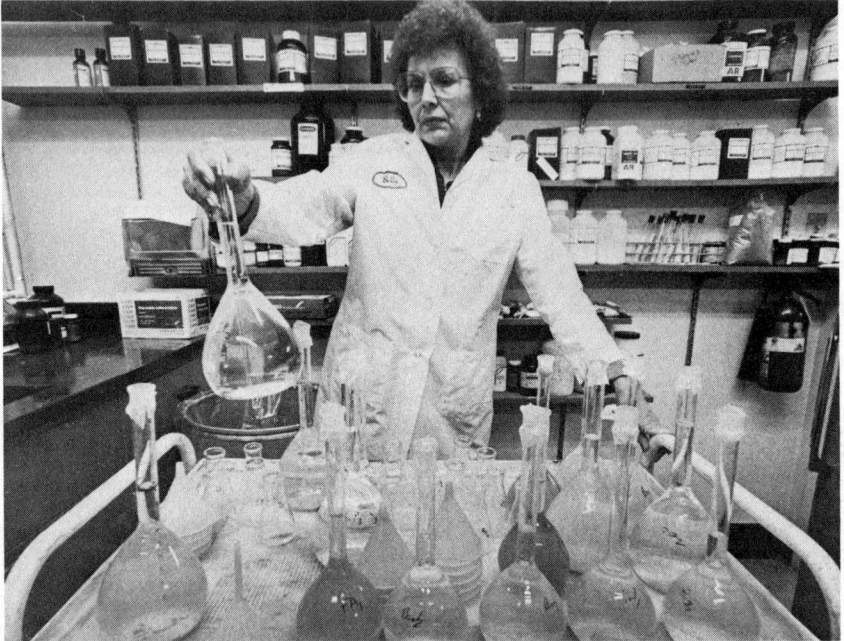

Liquified vitamin samples undergo many tests.

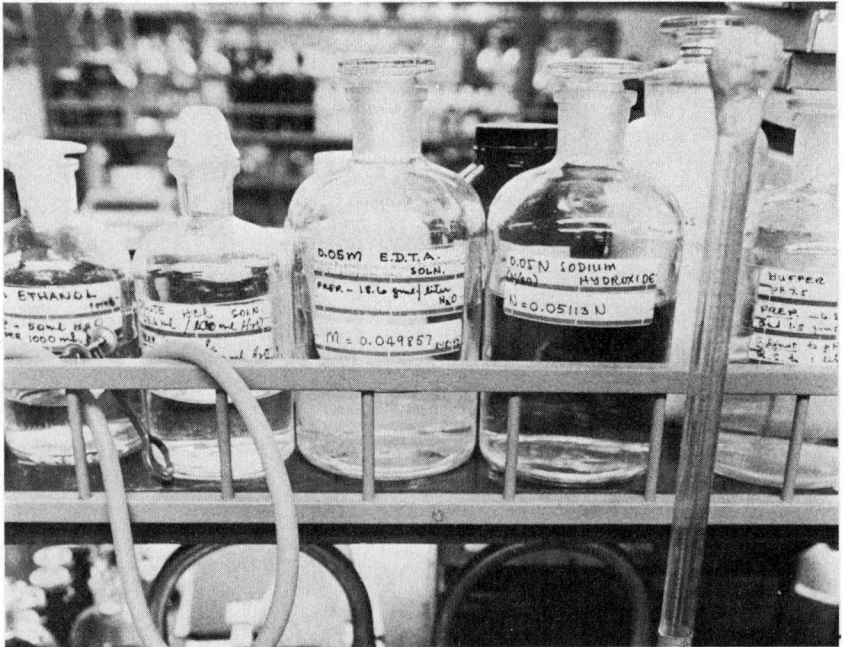

Vitamins are tested in the quality control lab.

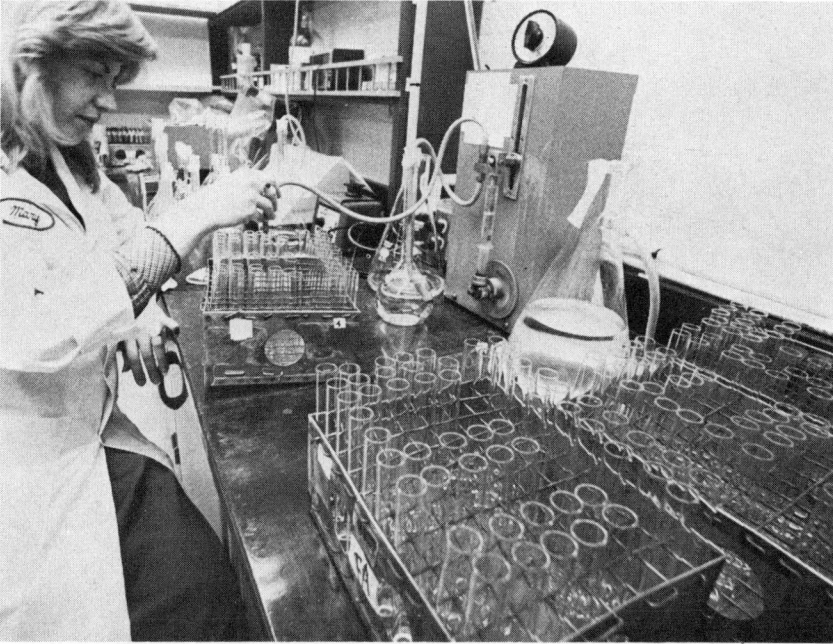

Here vitamins are tested for solubility.

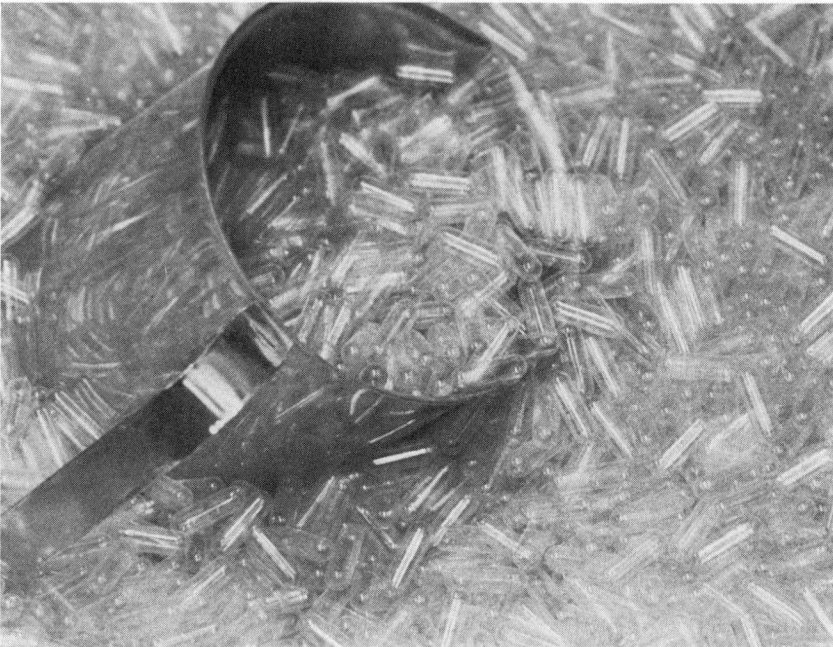

Thousands of empty capsules are used for vitamin containers.

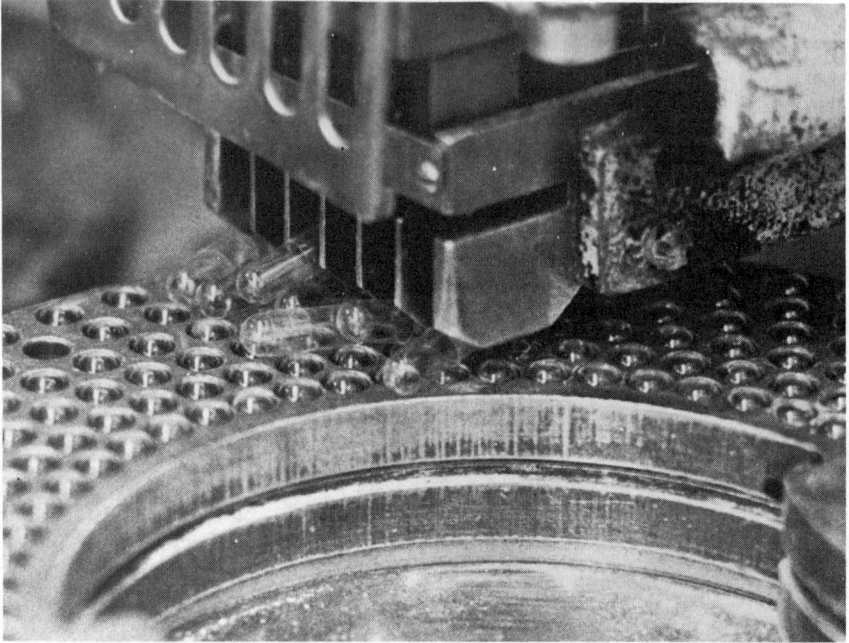

Emcapsulation machine readies capsules to receive their ingredients.

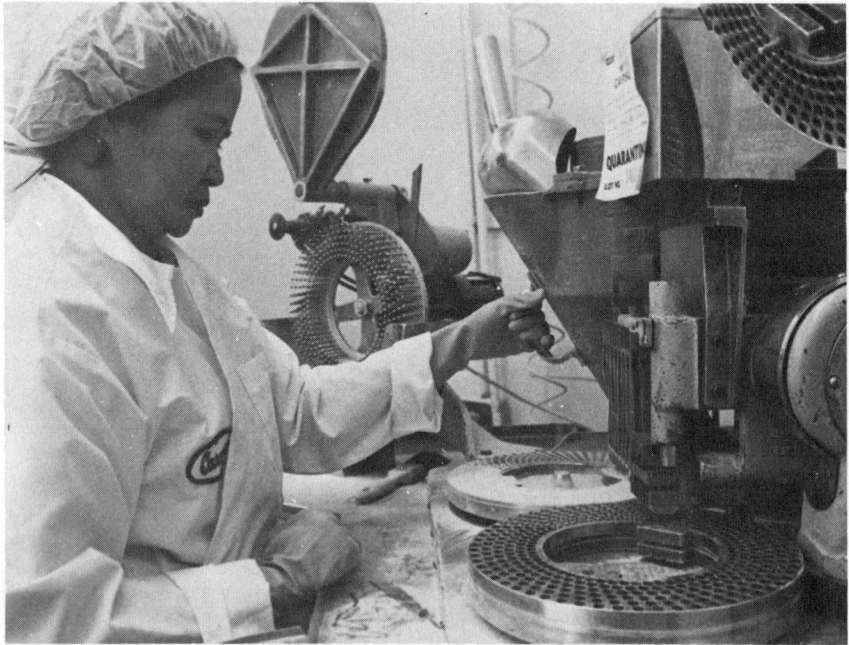

Vitamin material fills the capsules.

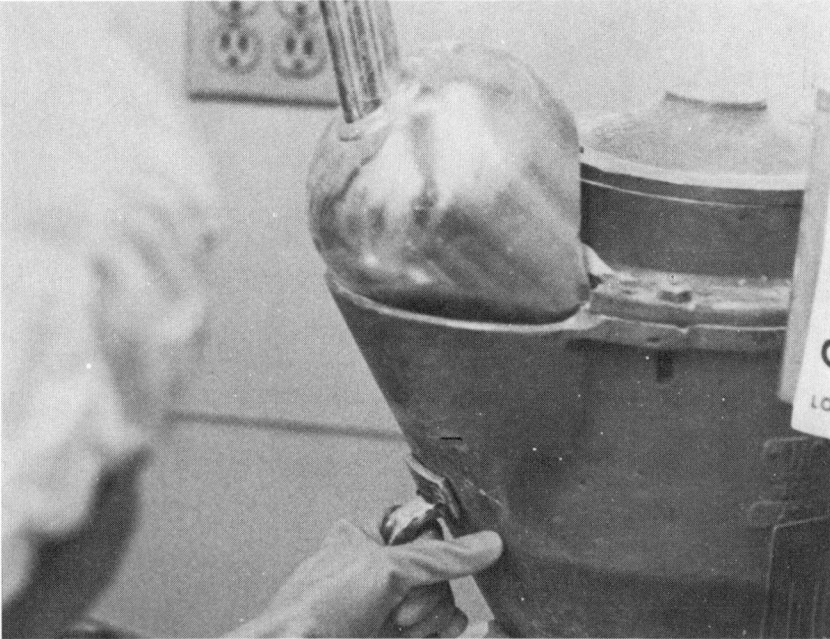

Thousands of capsules are filled with the vitamin mixture.

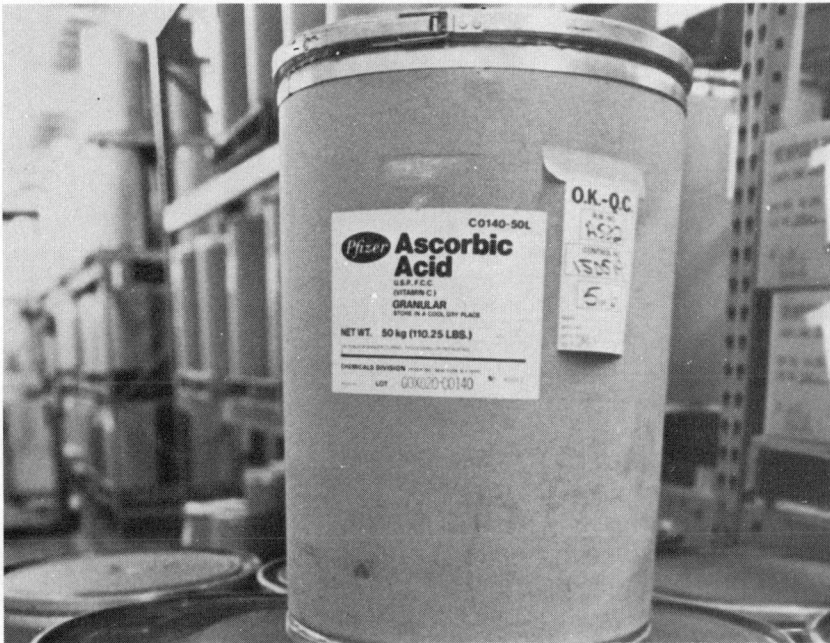

A 110-pound container holds vitamin C in the granular form.

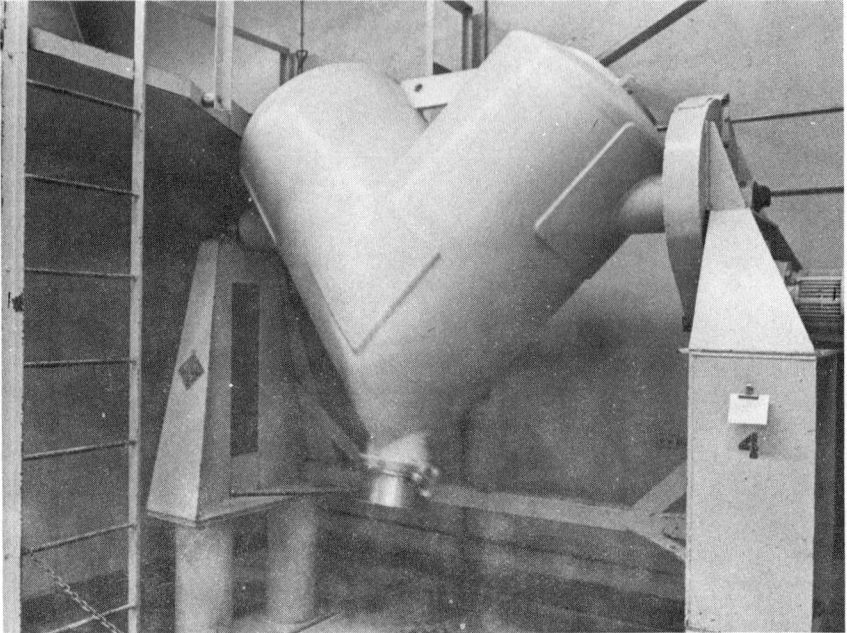

The first step in making a vitamin tablet is to sift the raw material into a V-blender.

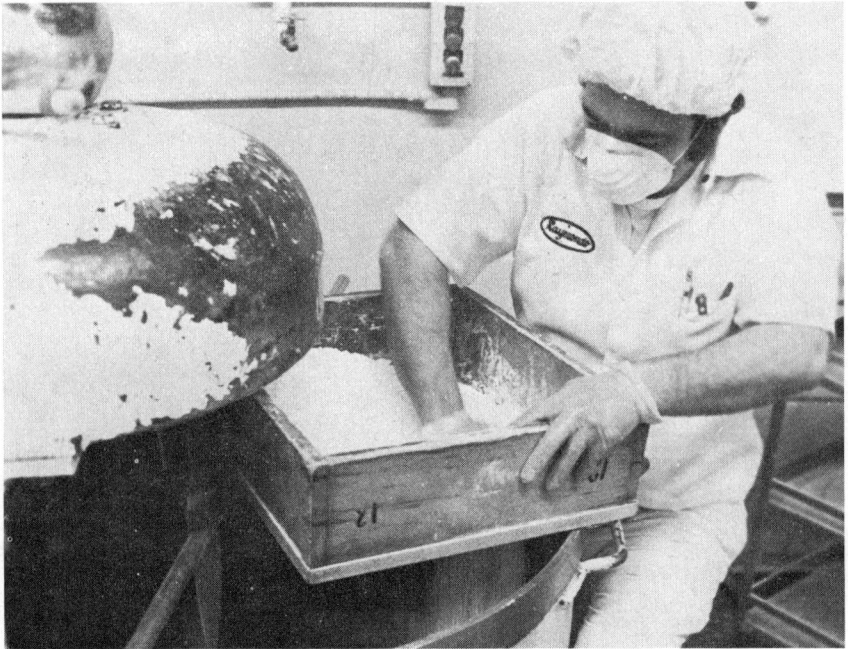

Raw materials are sifted in the granulating process.

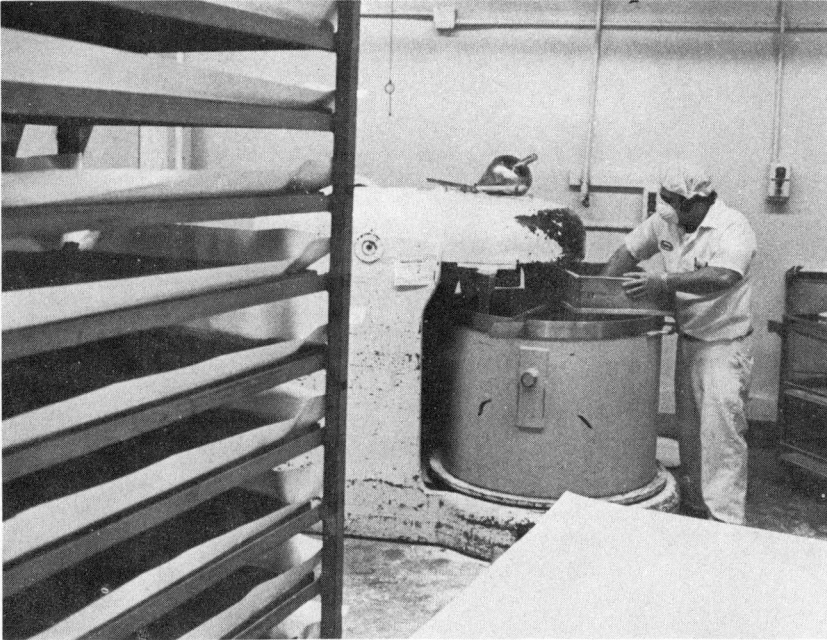

Once the raw materials are blended, they are placed on shelves to dry before being molded into tablets.

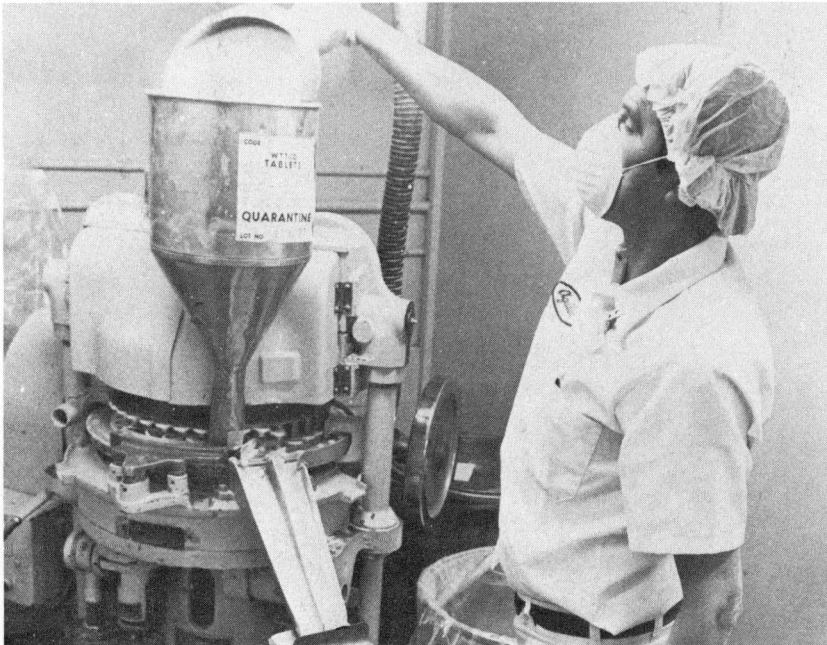

This machine compresses the material into tablet-form.

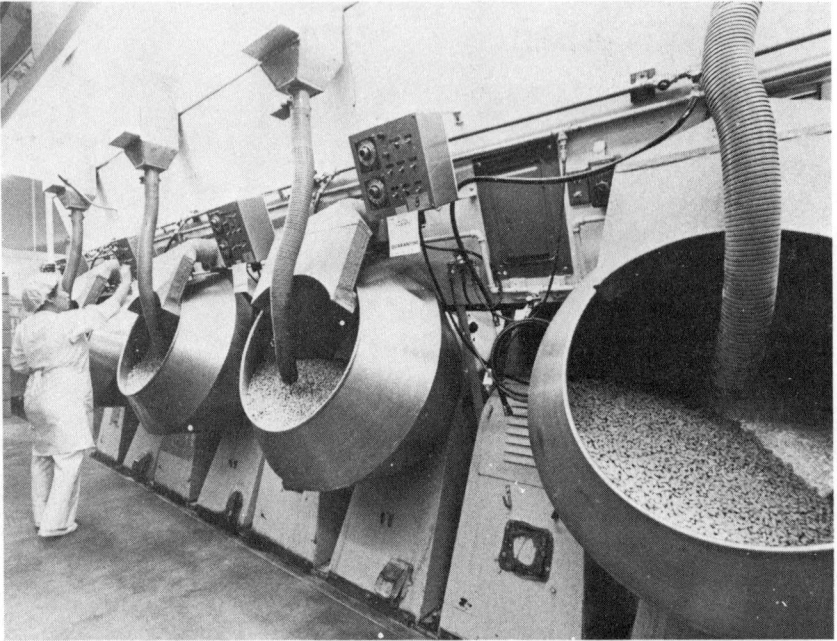

Vitamin tablets here are given a protective coating before bottling.

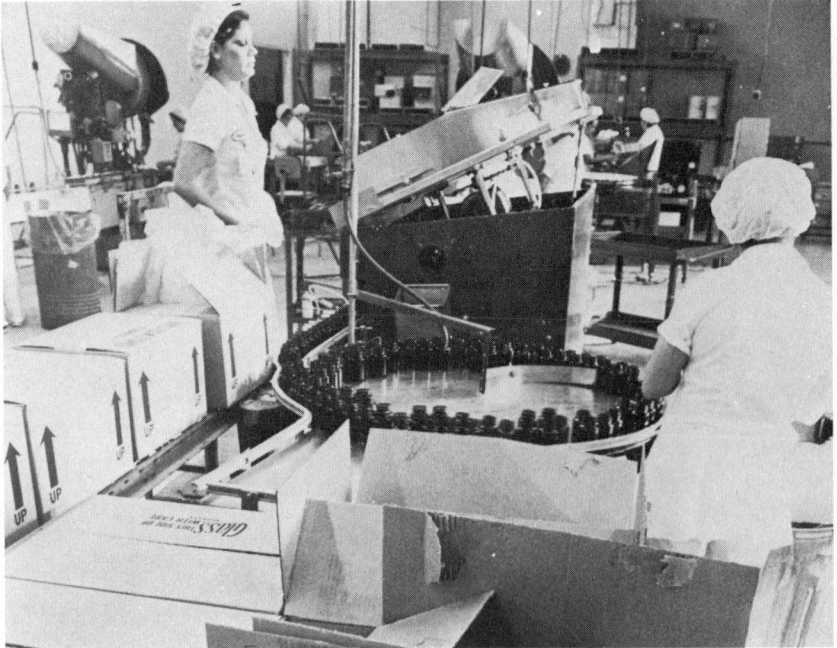

Once the tablets are made, the bottling process begins.

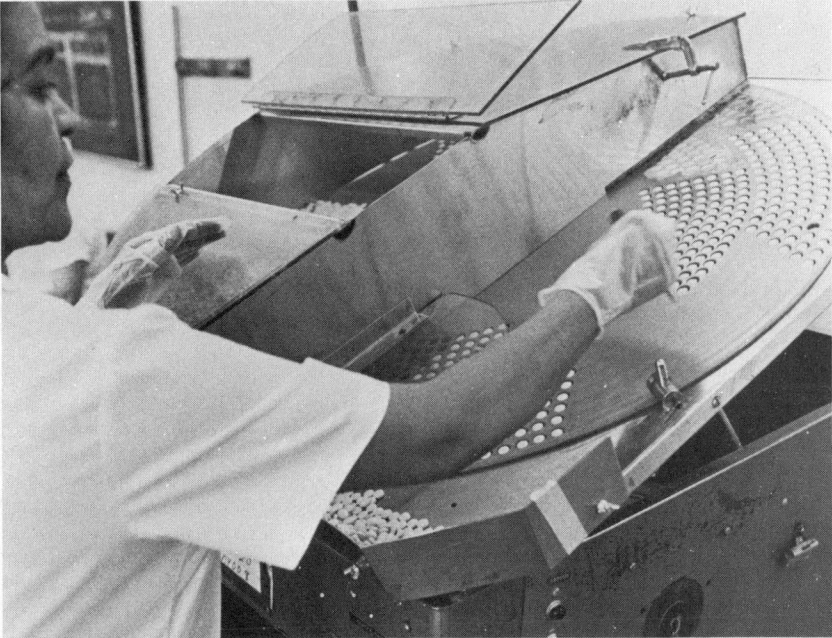

The automatic tablet-counting machine assures the consumer that he is receiving the proper quantity.

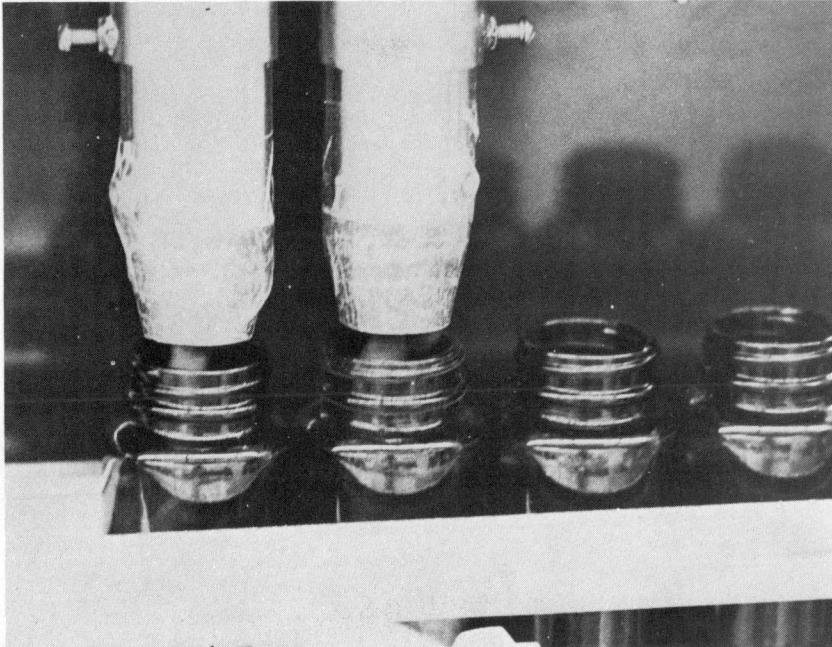

A close-up of the tablet-counting machine as tablets enter the bottles.

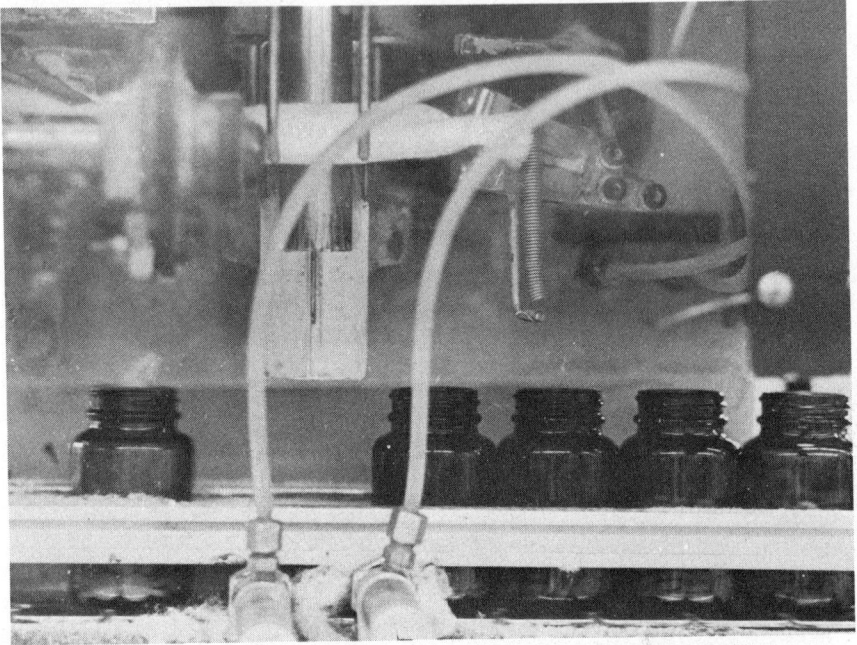

The bottles that have tablets move down the conveyer belt to the cotton-stuffing machine.

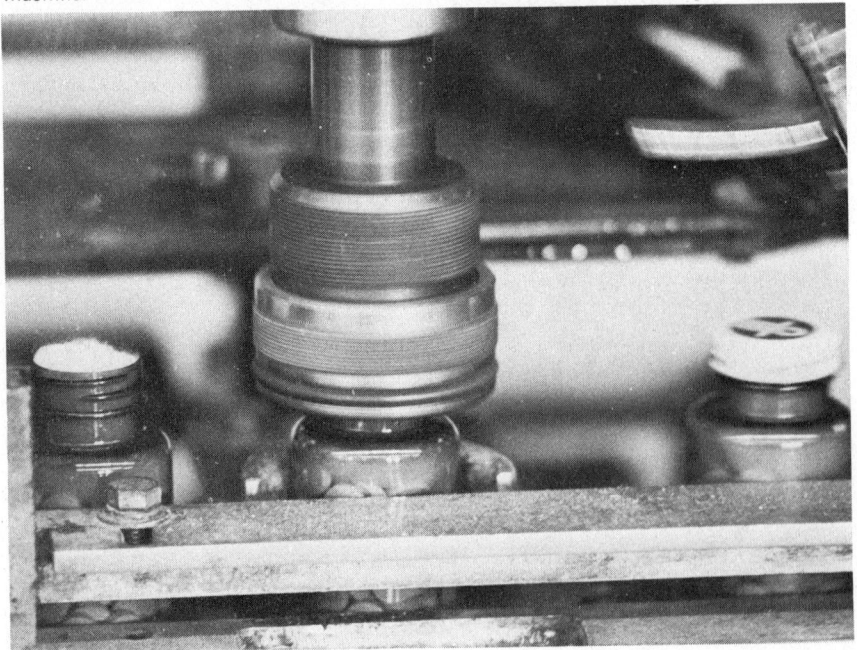

A machine then automatically screws on the caps.

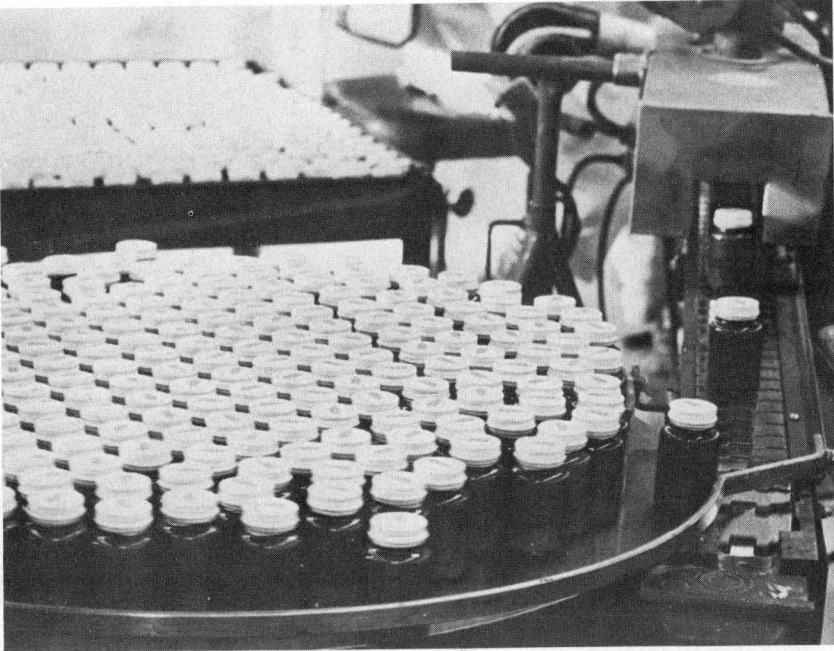

Hundreds of bottles, filled and stoppered, wait their turn on the conveyer belt for the final step, labeling.

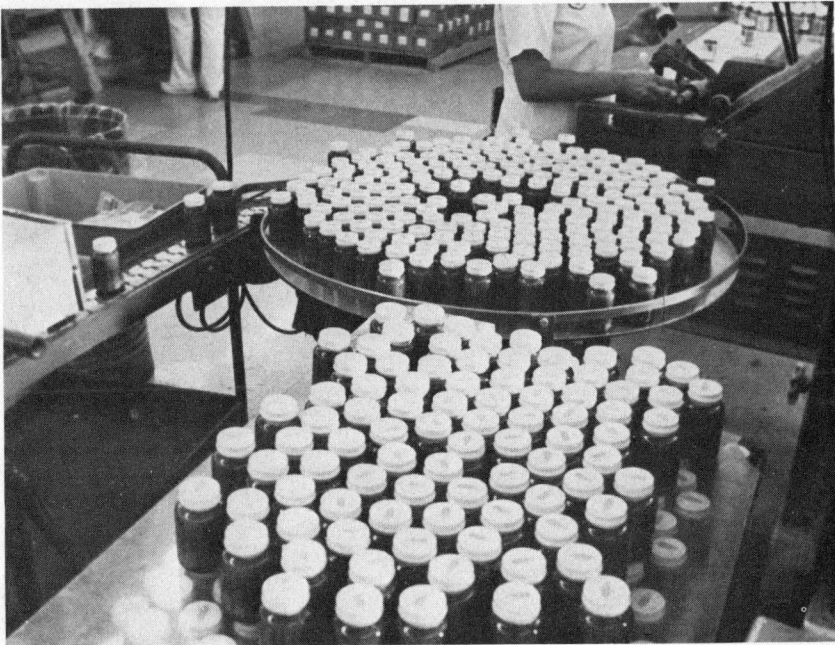

Bottles waiting for labels.

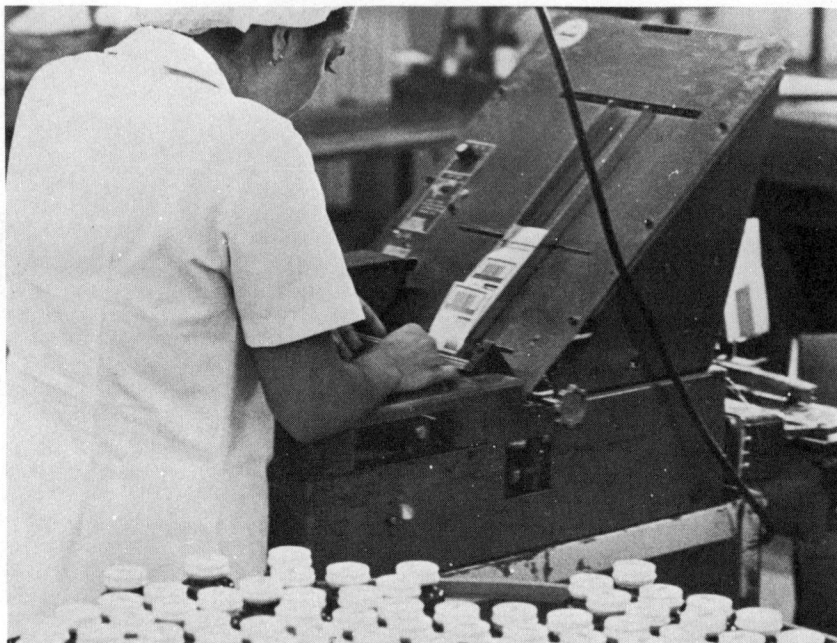

An employee mans the bottle labeling machine.

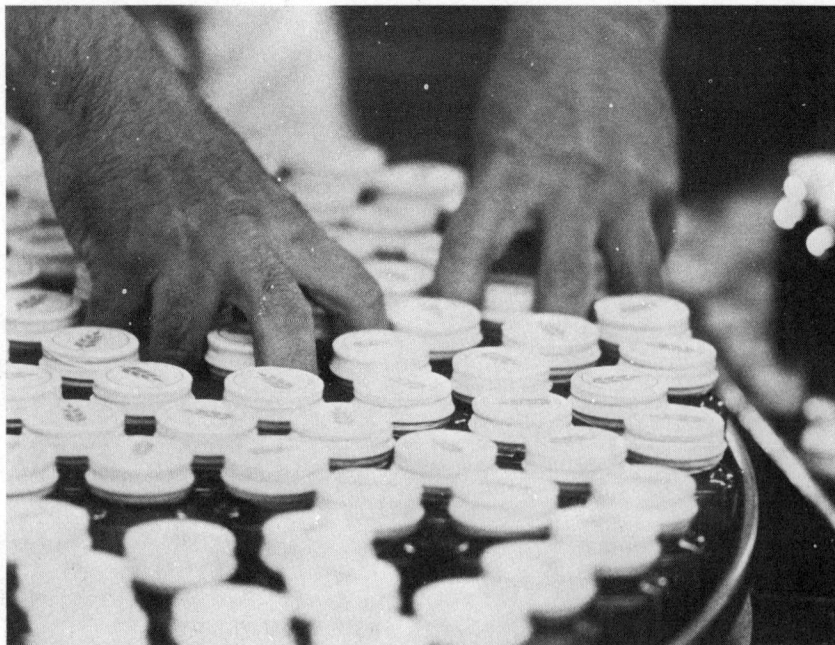

Bottles with labels on them are finally boxed for shipment.

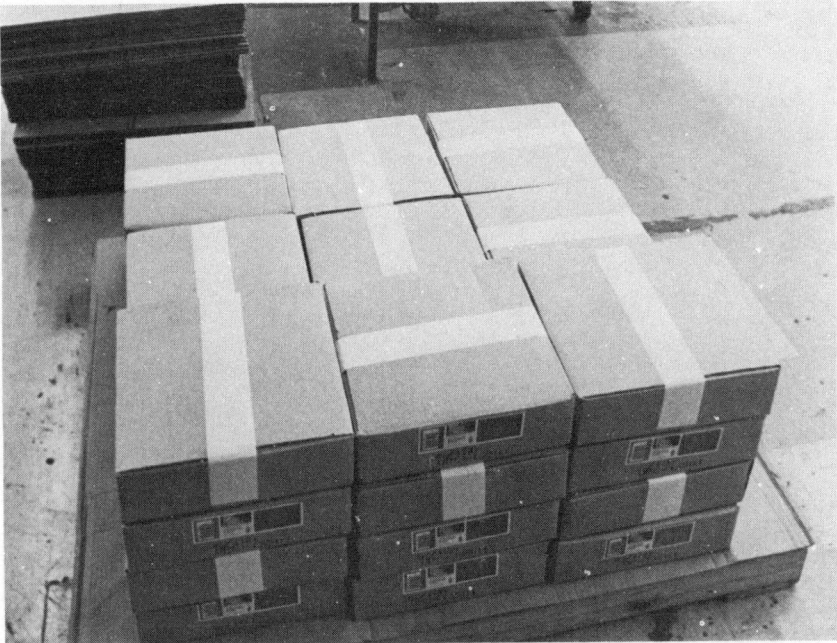

Boxed vitamins are stacked and readied for transport.

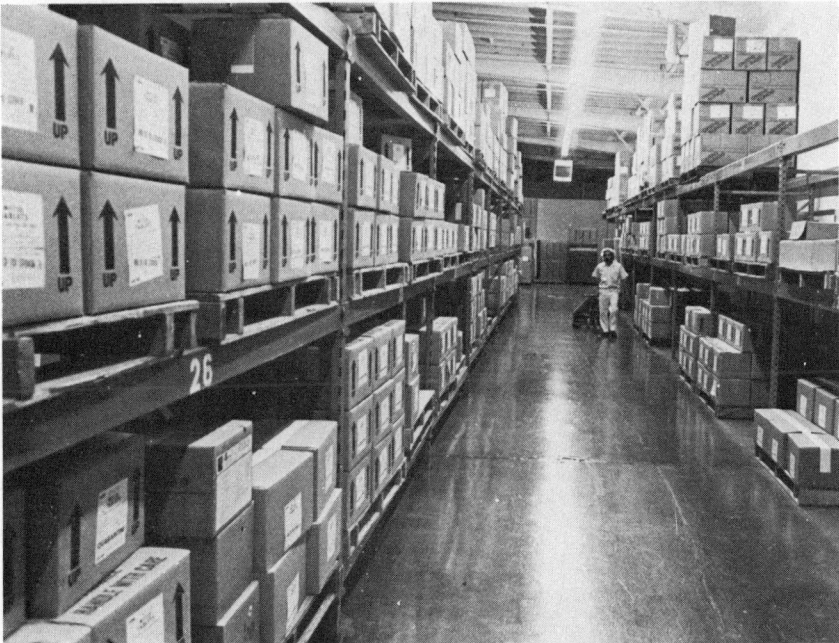

The vitamin warehouse of William T. Thompson Company.

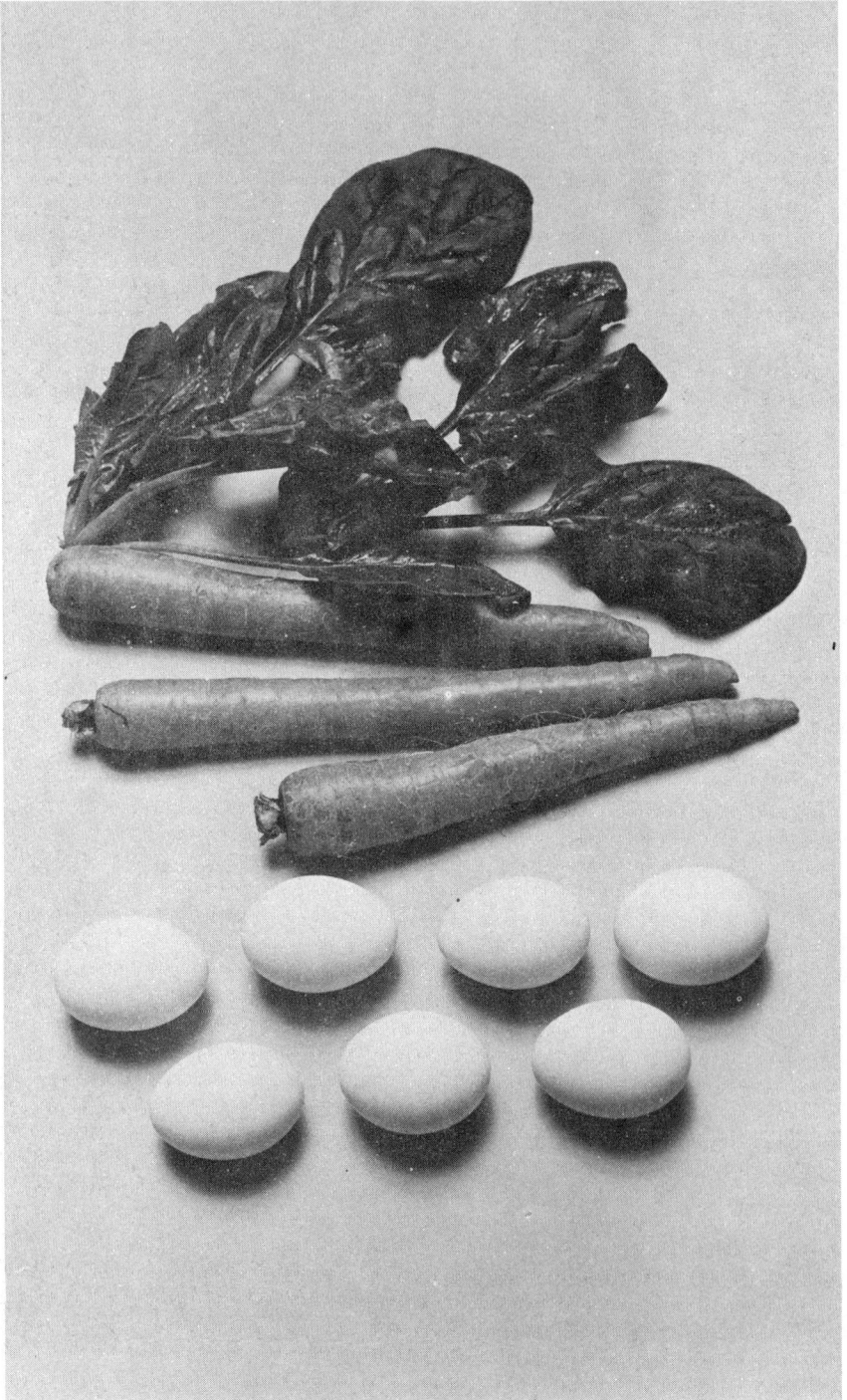

4

Vitamin A

FORM AND FUNCTION

In the alphabet soup of vitamins, A, of course, comes first, as did its discovery. Around 1913, at the University of Wisconsin, Elmer V. McCollum and Marguerite Davis found that adding milk fat or egg yolk to the purified diets of rats with stunted growth and eye lesions was enough to abate or reverse the symptoms. The effective substance, called Fat Soluble A by its discoverers, had the distinction of becoming the first vitamin and was isolated from cod-liver oil in 1937 and first synthesized in the lab in 1946.

Vitamin A exists in food in three preformed states (retinol, retinal, and retinoic acid), and in a precursor or provitamin state (carotene) that is converted to an active form in the body. Preformed A exists almost entirely in animal foods where animals store it—liver, kidneys and fat tissue—after converting it from carotene. Hence, it is abundant in organ meats and occurs in egg yolk, butter and whole dairy products. Most of the preformed A we get is the alcohol form called retinol, which occurs in foods and is stored in the body as retinyl esters (a compound of retinol and a fatty acid).

Most of us know provitamin A better as carotenes, the group of pigments that give carrots, squash, cantaloupes and fruits and other vegetables their yellow-orange color. However, carotenes, the most common form of which is beta-carotene, are also extremely prevalent in green plants whose chlorophyll hides their characteristic color. Once ingested, carotenes are converted to retinol by enzymes in the small intestine. After that change takes place, the body treats the carotene-derived A the same way as the preformed varieties. Both types are stored as retinyl esters in the

33

liver, kidneys, adrenal glands and adipose tissue. When needed by the body, the esters are converted to retinol, bound to a transport protein and made available to the tissues.

A is a versatile vitamin known to affect nearly every tissue in the body. As with all of the vitamins, our knowledge of it is just the tip of the iceberg, but one of its most important functions—and certainly one of its best understood—has to do with its role in vision. Retinal, which results from the oxidation of retinol released from the liver, combines with proteins called opsins to form special pigments in the photoreceptors—the rods and cones—of the eye. When light strikes these photoreceptors, the pigment (rhodopsin in the rods, which function in dim light, iodopsin in the cones, which function in bright light) splits into its component parts (retinal and opsin), transforming the visual signal into a nerve impulse that is sent to the brain by way of the optic nerve. Both the rods and the cones require vitamin A to perform their visual function, but the rods are more sensitive to its absence. Thus, a deficiency of vitamin A results in night blindness (nyctalopia), poor vision in dim light.

Night blindness, which is claimed by some to affect as much as one-third of the American population, can be corrected with vitamin A supplementation, but prolonged deficiency can lead to total blindness. Vitamin A deficiency is thought, in fact, to be the major cause of blindness in impoverished countries. Vitamin A's role in healthy vision is twofold, however, since it is necessary to maintain the structure of eye tissues.

Scientists have known for many years that vitamin A is necessary for normal growth and repair of epithelial cells, those that line the respiratory, digestive and reproductive tracts and form the outer layers of the skin. It is thought that vitamin A may perform this function by participating in the synthesis of substances in mucus and other secretions that lubricate and preserve the tissues and protect them against invasion by bacteria and other microorganisms. In the absence of A, epithelial cells slowly dry and harden, making the membranes less resistant to infection.

The big jobs of sight and cell maintenance aside, vitamin A is also involved in the ongoing process of developing and maintaining bones and teeth, and in synthesizing adrenal and thyroid hormones and possibly the steroid hormones necessary to reproduction.

DEFICIENCY

As mentioned, night blindness is usually the first sign of vitamin

A deficiency. Humans may also experience reduced resistance to infection (particularly of the eyes, ears, reproductive and respiratory tracts), eye inflammation, and rough, dry skin. This dry, hardened condition of the skin (keratinization) is particularly harmful to eye tissue and can eventually result in blindness, but it can also affect most of the body's surfaces, including the taste buds. Chronic diarrhea may result from changes in the digestive tract and nerve and bone changes may occur. A deficiency in children can result in stunted growth and damage to the central nervous system.

While deficiency symptoms are generally caused by a primary deficiency (insufficient dietary intake), vitamin A and the other fat-soluble vitamins are absorbed in much the same way fats are, so, as Dr. Patricia Kreutler notes, "Secondary deficiencies may be precipitated by absorptive disorders, including those caused by long-term use of mineral oil or prescribed drugs (that bind bile salts—author), or those caused by pancreatic or gall bladder disease, generally interfering with lipid metabolism." Vitamin A is also affected by liver disease such as hepatitis and by cystic fibrosis, which causes poor absorption of dietary fat and fat-soluble vitamins. Because vitamin A requires protein for transport to the tissues, protein deficiency has a negative effect on the vitamin's status.

WHAT CAN IT DO?

There is no end to the things vitamin A proponents say it can cure, from acne to hyperactivity. As with all the vitamins, these claims are often embroideries upon the functions the vitamin is known to perform in the body. Vitamin A, for example, is known to help maintain the epithelial cells, which line the skin. Thus, the vitamin purveyor will promote A as the vitamin that gives you a beautiful complexion. As you might guess, Americans go for it in a big way. Because A promotes bone growth, and a severe deficiency can lead to stunted growth in children, a conscientious mother, using the same kind of logic, might feed her child large doses of supplements to assure he grows up taller than his five feet eight father. Not only is such thinking fallacious, it can also be downright dangerous, as we'll learn when we talk about vitamin A's toxicity.

Despite claims, there is no scientific evidence to support vitamin A's use as a treatment for schizophrenia, learning disabilities or hyperactivity in children.

Doses of vitamin A ranging from 50,000 to 150,000 IU per day have been used in the treatment of acne, but the American Academy of Pediatrics has found that the beneficial effects of such treatment are neither consistent nor long-lasting. The FDA's Advisory Panel on Vitamin and Mineral Drug Products for Over-the-Counter Human Use came to the same conclusion in 1979. Further, they found A to be of no value in the treatment of the majority of eye, skin and respiratory diseases, since very few of these stem from a deficiency of the vitamin. A, is, of course, effective against night blindness and xeropthalmia (an eye disease in which the cornea and conjunctiva become dry and rough; it can result in total blindness if untreated), which are vitamin A deficiency diseases.

There is hope that a synthetic member of the vitamin A family, 13-cis-retinoic acid, may prove effective against very severe acne. The National Cancer Institute, testing the drug against cancer, used it to treat fourteen people with acne who had not been helped by any other medication. Although the results were dramatic, there were also numerous side effects. Still undergoing testing, the drug is not currently available to the public. Further, the FDA warns, "Even though some of the drugs used for acne are related to vitamin A, doctors warn that you should not try to treat yourself with large amounts of vitamin A that you can buy in drugstores or health food stores. Such self-treatment could lead to serious side effects, including damage to your liver." In *Nutrition In Perspective*, Dr. Patricia A. Kreutler also warns, "The drug is still classified as experimental; moreover, caution about its teratogenic effects (capability of causing fetus malformation) is advised. The new drug could not, for example, safely be given to women who are pregnant or not using some method of contraception, because it is one of a class of substances known to injure embryos."

This and other retinoids—synthetic forms of A or vitamin A analogues—are, however, currently at the forefront of some very promising cancer research. As we already know, vitamin A is necessary for the normal growth and repair of epithelial cells—those that line the lungs, bladder, breast, intestines, skin and many other organs where cancers frequently occur. Tests with laboratory animals have shown vitamin A to play a role in arresting or preventing malignant changes in epithelial tissue; large doses have even been reported to reverse tumor growth in some instances. Another study showed bronchial cancer patients to have significantly lower plasma vitamin A concentrations than controls. It has been suggested, however, that the lower concentrations of the vitamin may be the *result* of the disease rather than its cause. According to an official statement of the National Cancer Institute, "The effectiveness of vitamin A and its analogues as active chemopreventive agents for common forms of epithelial cancer has been demonstrated in animals. Vitamin A analogues have also been introduced into clinical trials. If their effectiveness in human patients is substantiated, it is possible that vitamin A analogues may be of benefit in delaying or preventing cancer, especially in high-risk groups."

Robert J. Avery, Jr. of the NCI indicated that clinical trials—those with human beings—of the A analogues are really just beginning. According to Avery, "Synthetic retinoids will be tested in two populations at high risk of developing cancer: women whose Pap tests indicate they have cervical dysplasia will receive retinal acetate in the form of a vaginal salve, and albinos who live in the intense sunlight of equatorial Africa and are at a high risk of developing skin cancer will receive an oral preparation containing a retinoid that may protect them from the damaging effects of ultraviolet light. Details of these trials are still being developed. It should be emphasized that therapy with synthetic retinoids is still considered investigational and, as yet, is of no proven benefit against cancer."

The vitamin A analogues being used in cancer research were developed, of course, because of the harmful side effects that occur when vitamin A is administered in doses large enough to be effective. It must be pointed out, however, that while vitamin A analogues are distributed differently in the body than the natural form and are considerably less toxic to the liver, there is still a critical lack of substantial clinical human data on these powerful drugs. The lack of such data precludes their general use at this time and these synthetic forms are not available to the public. As Dr. Kreutler points out, the "vitamin A supplements currently on the market are not known to have any cancer-preventing effect." Considering the potentially dangerous side effects associated with megadoses of vitamin A and its still very tentative role in cancer prevention, it is strongly advised that no one take the vitamin in quantities greatly exceeding the RDA.

TOXICITY

As a fat-soluble vitamin, A is stored by the body—primarily in the liver—and has the potential to build up to toxic levels when taken in excess. It must be pointed out, however, that only pre-formed vitamin A—that found in animal sources and supple-ments—is toxic, you cannot poison yourself on the provitamin A or carotene that is found in fruit and vegetable sources. The body will not convert carotene to retinol when it has enough.

The U.S. RDA for vitamin A is 1000 RE (5000 IU). Dr. Kreutler recommends that no more than 2000 RE (a very conservative rec-ommendation) be taken without medical recommendation and supervision. Yet many companies manufacture supplements con-taining 25,000 IU of vitamin A; the literature of one company states, "Serious scientists who have studied *real* nutritional needs have determined that man probably needs about 35,000 IU of vitamin A per day. Assuming at least a moderate dietary intake, a dosage form of 25,000 IU makes sense." But one wonders who those "serious scientists" are, because those concerned with public health and safety find continued doses of five to ten times the RDA very risky.

Ironically, as with some of the other potentially toxic vitamins, the beginning signs of toxicity for vitamin A are the same as those for a deficiency. It isn't uncommon for self-prescribing individuals to misinterpret the symptoms and dose themselves even more heavily with substances already causing a toxic reaction. The list of symptoms associated with hypervitaminosis A is long and ser-ious: headache, nausea, diarrhea, irritability, blurred vision, ringing in the ears, dry, cracked skin and mucous membranes, hair loss, brittle nails, enlargement of the liver and spleen, bone, joint, mus-cle and abdomen pain, menstrual problems, and pressure within the skull that mimics a brain tumor. Megadoses of vitamin A can be particularly serious for pregnant and lactating women, as well as for infants. High A intakes have been linked to various birth defects; and children fed large supplements are subject to stunted growth, hydrocephalus (water on the brain) and other disorders.

Yet, despite the very serious—and fairly well-publicized—impli-cations for vitamin A overdose, Kreutler reports that "hypervita-minosis A has been on the increase in recent years, with numerous reports of intakes in the range of 25,000 to 100,000 IU per day. Such quantities present a real risk to health, especially to pregnant women and the fetus." Jane Brody, too, makes a telling comment about our recent infatuation with megadosing: "With so many people taking megadoses of vitamins, poisonous excesses of one or another fat-soluble vitamin may become as common a medical problem as deficiencies."

RDA AND AVAILABILITY

The RDA for vitamin A is 1000 RE (5000 IU) for males over eleven, 800 RE (4000 IU) for women of the same age. Vitamin A and its precursor carotene are freely available in foods, making it extremely unlikely that any normal, healthy person consuming an adequate diet should face a deficiency. Among the best food sources are liver, green and most orange-yellow fruits and vegetables, eggs and whole milk. Most of us get about half our vitamin A in the active form from animal foods and convert the other half from the carotene in fruits and vegetables. Fried beef liver, an excellent source, provides approximately 45,000 IU of the vitamin in a single serving. Livers of all types, as well as the commonly administered fish liver oils, are extremely potent sources of the vitamin, which leads to a word of caution. A is one of the rare vitamins of which you can get an excess in foods, as a couple of over-zealous mothers recently learned by feeding their babies daily rations of chopped livers instead of "nutritionally deficient" commercial baby foods. Both children suffered the serious side effects of vitamin A overdose. As already mentioned, you cannot poison yourself on the provitamin A in plant foods (though your skin may take on a yellow cast if the intake is high enough), but livers and fish liver oils can be another story if consumed in overabundance. Because the body stores vitamin A, a serving of liver supplies enough of the vitamin for about nine days. Reserves are also sufficient to make daily intake of the vitamin unnecessary.

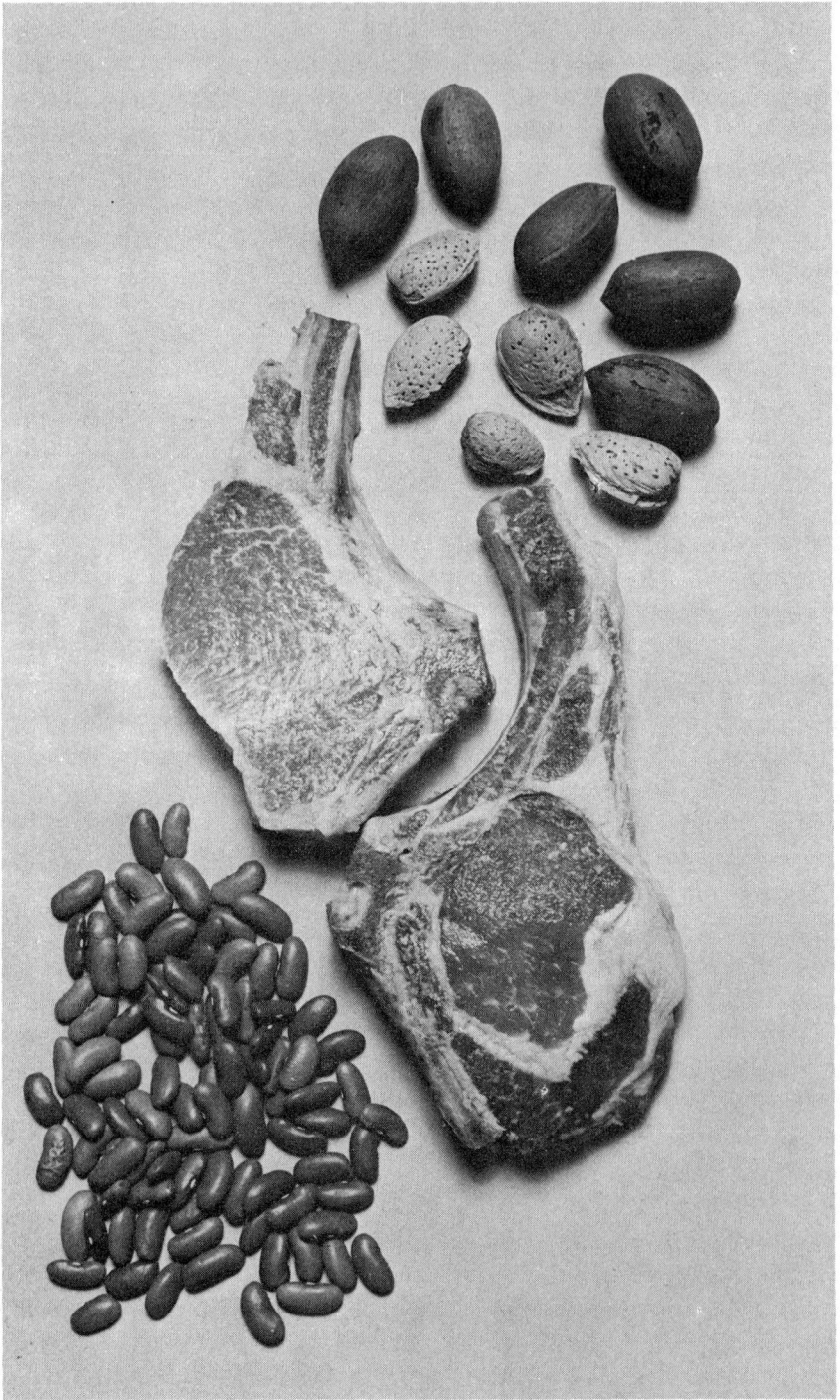

5

Thiamin (B1)

FORM AND FUNCTION

All of the vitamins that form the B-complex are water-soluble and function as components of coenzymes necessary to catalyze the body's many biochemical reactions. The majority of the Bs, namely thiamin, riboflavin, niacin, biotin and pantothenic acid, are involved in converting the food we eat into energy. Because they are water-soluble, the B vitamins are capable of very limited storage in the body, with the excess being flushed out daily in the urine.

Thiamin is a busy B that plays a part in at least 20 different enzyme reactions that metabolize dietary fats, proteins and carbohydrates. A number of researchers were on the trail of thiamin before Casimir Funk was credited with its discovery in 1912. Among these was a medical officer in the Japanese Navy in the mid-1880s who was concerned with the prevalence among sailors on long voyages of beriberi, a disease characterized by extreme weakness, numbness and paralysis, anemia and wasting away. Takaki, who felt the key to the disease lay in the crews' diets of polished rice (that with the husk and bran stripped away), added milk and meat to the daily regimens of those at sea. The good doctor's hunch was correct; only those sailors who turned down the new rations were afflicted with beriberi.

A short time later, a Dutch physician, Christiaan Eijkman, noticed that chickens fed a steady diet of polished rice developed the symptoms of beriberi, and that feeding unpolished rice made the symptoms disappear. Further experiments elicited the same results in human subjects. In 1901 nutrition researcher Gerrit Grijns put

41

forth the theory that unpolished rice contained an unknown substance that prevented beriberi. The vitamin was finally synthesized in 1936. The discovery of the thiamin/beriberi link effectively put an end to a disease of epidemic proportions that virtually did not exist prior to the technology that allowed man to polish rice and refine wholesome grains into white flour of considerably lower nutritional value.

Funk named the new-found substance for its sulfur content (from *thio*, the Greek for sulfur) and for its amine group. As we already know, based on his knowledge of thiamin(e), he assumed all of the "accessory factors" found in foods contained amines; hence, the term "vitamine" was coined.

But thiamin is noteworthy for more than lending an erroneous name to a new class of nutrients. Thiamin is absorbed in the small intestine where it is transformed into its active form, thiamin pyrophosphate. As Kreutler notes, this coenzyme form "is crucial to the energy-generating reactions involving carbohydrates, fatty acids, and amino acids." In effect, without the help of thiamin, the food we eat could not be converted into the energy that gets us through our daily deeds. In its spare time, thiamin also participates in the metabolism of nucleic acids and in converting the amino acid tryptophan to the B vitamin niacin. When an extra phosphate is added to thiamin it becomes thiamin triphosphate, which is suspected to be a component of nerve cell membranes and to function in the transmission of nerve impulses.

Very little thiamin is stored in the body; about half of it resides in muscle tissue, the remainder in the major organs. The body requires a daily intake of thiamin, as these small stores are rapidly depleted.

DEFICIENCY

The initial symptoms of thiamin deficiency include loss of appetite, nausea, heart problems, spastic muscle contractions, mental confusion, low morale, edema (swelling due to an accumulation of fluid in the body), impaired growth and wasting of tissues. Prolonged deficiency leads, of course, to beriberi, a comical-sounding disease with a not so comical progression of symptoms that can end in death. For those who have always wondered about the name, *beri* means "weakness" in Singhalese, the language of the principal race of Ceylon. There is definitely enough weakness connected with the disease—which strikes in three forms: wet, dry and infantile—to warrant repeating it twice.

In underdeveloped countries a diet of polished rice is most often the culprit in a thiamin deficiency that leads to beriberi; in places like the U.S. the disease, which can lead to permanent brain damage, is more likely to be a result of chronic alcoholism. Not only do alcoholics usually subsist on sorely inadequate diets, but alcohol itself interferes with the absorption of all the B vitamins. Other nemeses to this nutrient include barbiturates, alkaline substances (antacids, bicarbonate of soda, etc.), and diuretics. Those particularly susceptible to deficiencies include pregnant and lactating women and the elderly.

WHAT CAN IT DO?

At the present time, about all thiamin is known to do is prevent or cure clinical or sub-clinical beriberi; only your doctor can tell you if the symptoms you are experiencing (perhaps nausea, weakness, mental confusion, etc.) are due to a thiamin deficiency. Like most of the B vitamins, thiamin is often touted to give you more energy. While involved in the conversion of food to energy, thiamin alone contains no miracle energy-producing capabilities. It needs food on which to work; and taking in a wide variety of food is, under normal circumstances, enough to ensure plenty of thiamin to help process it, as well.

Other powers with which thiamin has been invested are those to prevent motion sickness and repel mosquitoes. Neither claim has been substantiated. Further, it is claimed to be beneficial in the treatment of such diseases as dermatitis, multiple sclerosis, neuritis and mental disorders. As *The Vitamin Book* by the Editors of Consumer Guide notes, "The Advisory Panel on Vitamin and Mineral Drug Products for Over-The-Counter Human Use concluded that thiamin supplements are of no benefit in the treatment of any of these symptoms or diseases in which there is no evidence of a thiamin deficiency."

TOXICITY

While hypersensitivity may be associated with excessive amounts of thiamin (particularly when taken intravenously), megadosing appears to be relatively safe. K.C. Hayes and D. Mark Hegsted conclude that this "is probably due to the fact that 5 mg is the maximum quantity that can be absorbed from a given dose." Quantities above and beyond that are carried out of the body in the urine, adversely affecting nothing, it seems, aside from the consumer's pocketbook.

RDA AND AVAILABILITY

The amount of thiamin each individual requires is actually determined by his diet. The more food a person eats, the more thiamin he needs to metabolize it. A high-carbohydrate diet makes greater thiamin demands than does one where fats and proteins predominate, but many foods rich in complex carbohydrates contain adequate supplies of thiamin, so additional intake of the vitamin is almost automatic. The RDAs are based on an estimated optimal intake of 0.5 mg of thiamin per 1000 calories. Thus, the recommended allowance is 1.4 mg for men between the ages of 23 and 50, and 1.0 mg for women of the same age.

Because thiamin does not occur in large quantities in most foods—brewer's yeast and pork are notable exceptions—it is fortunate that it appears in a great number of them, making RDAs relatively easy to meet. Other rich sources are nuts, seeds, legumes, brown rice, and whole-grain products of all types. Thiamin is also one of the few nutrients added back to refined grain products, so enriched breads and cereals are also adequate sources. While vegetables and fruits are already a rather poor source of thiamin, dried fruits contain virtually none of the vitamin, which is destroyed by the sulfur dioxide used in processing. Possessing the fragility of the other B vitamins, thiamin is easily lost in processing of all kinds and in cooking.

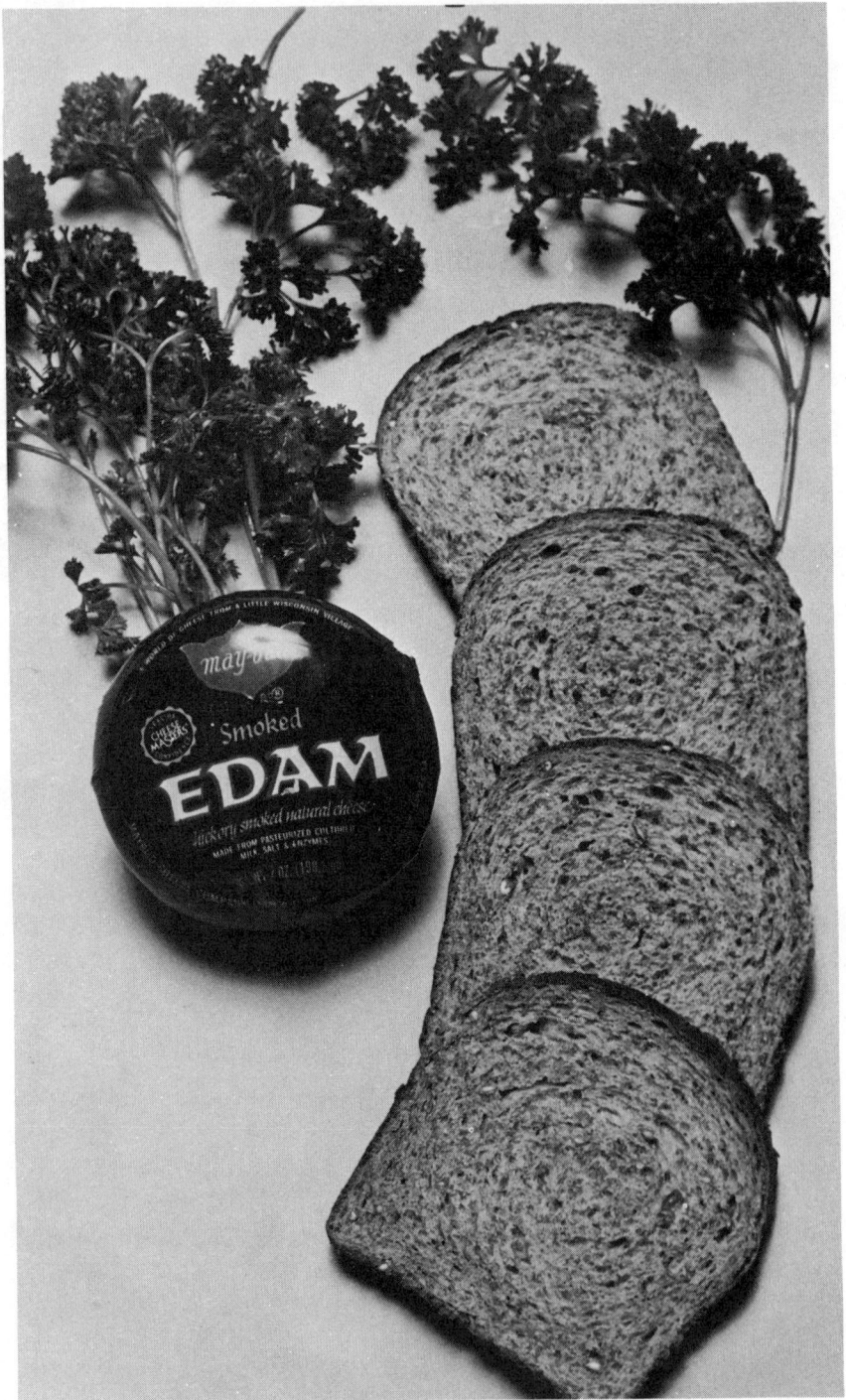

6

Riboflavin (B2)

FORM AND FUNCTION

The discovery of riboflavin essentially came from two different directions: from one group of scientists looking for a growth-promoting vitamin they believed to exist in foods even in the absence of thiamin, and from another group of researchers studying an energy-producing enzyme. When broken down, one part of the enzyme had something in common with the growth-promoting substance the vitamin-hunting scientists kept isolating: they were both yellow in color.

The yellow substance in both instances was riboflavin (*flavin* is from the Latin for "yellow"; *ribo* was pinned on the chemical group in the compound that resembled the pentose sugar d-ribose). The dual approach to the vitamin's discovery was one of the first indications to scientists of the way in which many B vitamins function as coenzymes in many of the body's energy-producing, growth-promoting chemical reactions. Originally tagged vitamin G, riboflavin became B2 for its similarity in chemical structure and dietary source to the first B vitamin, thiamin. It was successfully synthesized in the laboratory in 1935.

Phosphorus is added to riboflavin in the small intestine, where the vitamin is absorbed prior to transport to the liver with the aid of the water-soluble protein albumin. As with the other Bs, storage of riboflavin—primarily in the liver, kidneys and heart—is limited, although a sort of built-in safety factor seems to increase storage as intake of the vitamin decreases. Daily intake of riboflavin should be a dietary goal, as excesses are excreted in the urine. As Kreutler notes, "an even greater amount (of riboflavin) is found in the feces.

47

Fecal riboflavin originates not from metabolized food but from bacterial synthesis of the vitamin in the intestine. Whether riboflavin of intestinal origin is absorbed and metabolized for use by the body...and, if so, to what extent, is not known at present."

Riboflavin is active in two coenzyme forms: flavin mononucleotide or riboflavin monophosphate, and flavin adenine dinucleotide. Combined with proteins to form flavoproteins, these substances, like thiamin, are the little magicians that help transform food into energy. It is thought that riboflavin may also have a role in producing red blood cells and synthesizing particular hormones.

DEFICIENCY

A deficiency of riboflavin (called ariboflavinosis) alone is difficult to pinpoint since this vitamin works so closely with the other Bs. Lack of riboflavin has been indicted in stunted growth, but, again, this may be attributable to a lack of other vitamins, too. More easily blamed on riboflavin deficiency are such symptoms as inflamed mouth and lips with cracks at the corners, smooth, purple-tinted tongue, impaired vision and lesions of the cornea, dermatitis and itching, tearing and burning of the eyes.

WHAT CAN IT DO?

Basically, riboflavin can alleviate symptoms connected with, you guessed it, riboflavin deficiency. It cannot clear up the dozens of eye disorders not related to such a deficiency, and it's doubtful that widespread deficiency is the reason, as Ruth Adams suggests in *The Complete Home Guide To All The Vitamins*, "why so many folks must wear dark glasses these days." There is also no proof of riboflavin's usefulness in conjunction with the rest of the B-complex in megavitamin therapies for various ills. Neither is there anything in the literature to back up claims that it reduces sweet tooth or prevents insomnia.

TOXICITY

A report on the toxicity of riboflavin is short and sweet: megadosing has shown no adverse effects to date. As with all vitamins, however, and particularly the Bs, overconsumption of one can affect levels of others.

RDA AND AVAILABILITY

As with thiamin, the amount of riboflavin necessary in the diet is related to the number of calories consumed. Once determined by body size, recommended riboflavin levels are now determined by energy intake. Based on a figure of 0.60 mg per 1000 calories, the RDA for men 23 to 50 is 1.6 mg, for women in the same age group it is 1.2 mg.

A fine source of riboflavin is milk, which, by the glass, provides one-third of a woman's daily needs and one-fourth of a man's. Other dairy products do equally well; and those concerned about the fat content of their diet—as we all should be—can opt for the low- or non-fat variety, which have the added bonus of even more riboflavin than whole-milk products.

Riboflavin occurs in moderate amounts in a wide variety of foods; some of the best sources include meats—particularly liver and other organ meats—green, leafy vegetables, yeast and fortified grain products. As Rich Wentzler points out in his version of *The Vitamin Book*, "Vitamin B2 is also one of the lucky three vitamins that's put back into some of the grain products it's removed from. Not only that but they put back *more* than they take out, thanks to an early overestimate of wheat's riboflavin content." Thus, fortified breads and cereals are a much better source of the vitamin than are whole-grain ones. That, in a nutshell, may be the only nice thing that can be said about refined wheat products.

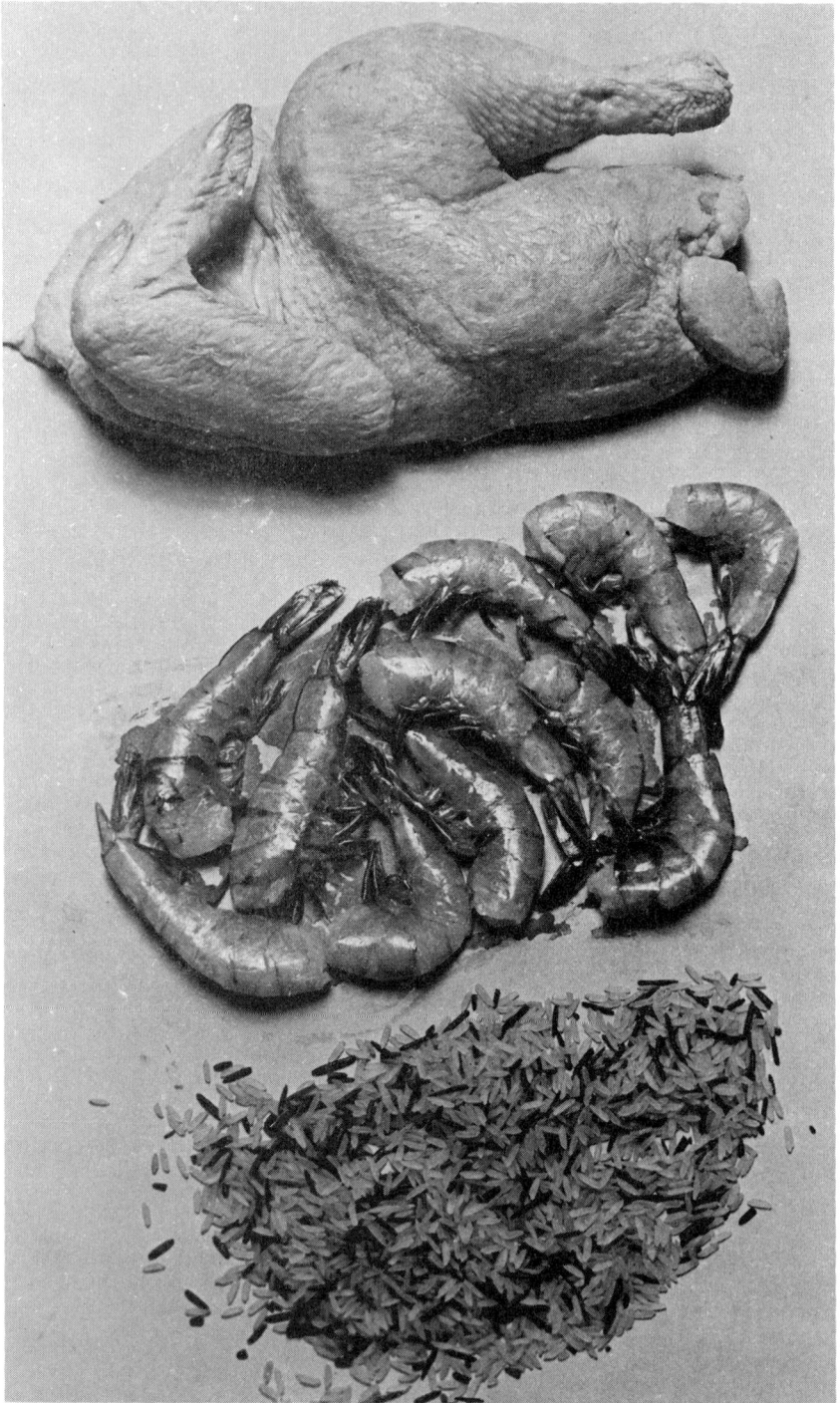

7

Niacin (B3)

FORM AND FUNCTION

References to a disease called pellagra (from the Italian for "rough skin"), first appeared in writing in 18th-century Spain and Italy. The disease, which is accompanied by severe dermatitis resembling burns, diarrhea, anorexia, and mental disturbance, had become commonplace in the Mediterranean countries after cornmeal introduced from the New World replaced wheat flour as a mainstay of the diet. In the early 20th century the U.S. saw its own serious outbreak of the disease—about 150,000 cases a year among the Southern poor who largely subsisted on a diet of cornmeal, molasses and fatty salt pork. Many cases of the disease showed up in the spring after an even more deficient winter diet.

Despite a rash of theories of all types—that pellagra was an infectious disease or one caused by spoiled corn, Joseph Goldberger, a doctor working for the U.S. Public Health Service in the South, believed the disease was linked to diet. He experimented first with children in an orphanage who suffered the disease, then volunteers from a prison farm in Mississippi. In both cases he found that adding milk, meat and yeast or eggs to the diet made the terrible symptoms disappear. The substance that did the trick was labeled the P-P (pellagra preventive) factor by Goldberger.

Meanwhile, researchers had known for some time about a compound called nicotinic acid, which had first been oxidized from nicotine in 1867. Funk had found it, too, in the rice polishings that were discovered to contain thiamin. In 1937 nicotinic acid and Goldberger's P-P factor were revealed to be one and the same when

51

Conrad Elvehjem, who is credited with the vitamin's discovery, found that the substance cured black tongue, a pellagra-like disease in dogs. The new vitamin's name was changed to niacin in 1971.

Niacin was, for a long time, surrounded by a number of unanswered questions. First, why was pellagra so closely associated with a diet based on cornmeal, since corn is actually quite rich in niacin? The answer is that the niacin in corn and some other grains is chemically bound in such a way that makes it unavailable to us. Mexicans and American Indians have long been onto something, as their custom of soaking corn in lime salts somehow makes the niacin content more readily available. Second, why was milk, which is very low in niacin, able to reverse pellagra's symptoms? Because, as Willard Krehl and others at the University of Wisconsin were to learn in 1945, the body is able to convert the amino acid tryptophan—in which milk is very rich—to niacin. The conversion, which requires the assistance of the B vitamins thiamin, riboflavin and pyridoxine, is accomplished at the rate of about 60 mg of dietary tryptophan to equal one milligram of niacin (one niacin equivalent). Kreutler states that the "estimated rate of conversion may not always be the same. For example, conversion is probably less efficient in people who consume diets low in niacin or low in tryptophan."

Niacin, which is absorbed in the upper portion of the small intestine, is, like the other Bs, stored in only small quantities in the body, making it necessary to take the vitamin in on a daily basis. Niacin above and beyond the body's daily need and tissue stores is excreted in the urine.

Niacin occurs in two forms in food: nicotinic acid and nicotinamide. The latter is the physiologically active form to which nicotinic acid is converted in the body. As a component of two coenzymes, nicotinamide adenine dinucleotide and nicotinamide adenine dinucleotide phosphate (which aren't names you'll be tossing around in conversation), niacin is an essential element in the process of metabolizing fats, proteins and carbohydrates...or converting food to energy.

DEFICIENCY

Pellagra, the niacin deficiency disease, is an insidious illness that often begins with indigestion, diarrhea, weight loss and weakness. One of its most characteristic symptoms is severe dermatitis resembling burns, where the skin is exposed to sunlight or irritation.

As Sue Rodwell Williams notes in *Nutrition and Diet Therapy*, infection often occurs as the skin lesions rupture and healing leaves darkly pigmented areas. Besides diarrhea and dermatitis, one of the other Ds in niacin deficiency is dementia. The mental disturbance that goes along with the disease can range from irritability, apathy, depression and confusion to delirium or insanity.

As with the other B vitamins, the deficiency disease associated with niacin is a complex reaction that may actually be linked to a shortage of several of the B vitamins. This is particularly true of niacin since it is known that B1, B2 and B6 are needed for the conversion of tryptophan to the vitamin. Thus, a shortage of any of these could result in a deficiency of niacin, as well. Large amounts of leucine (an amino acid) in the diet may also result in a deficiency, since this substance, as Kreutler observes, "either interferes with the synthesis of niacin from tryptophan or alters niacin metabolism in some other, as yet unidentified way."

Those most susceptible to a niacin deficiency are those taking drugs that interfere with its absorption, chronic alcoholics, or persons with amebic dysentery, hookworm or malaria.

WHAT CAN IT DO?

To treat pellagra, which can end in death if allowed to progress, as much as 25 to 50 mg of niacin a day is often administered. Because of the variety of symptoms associated with pellagra, particularly those relating to the nervous system, niacin has been promoted for the cure of a wide variety of ills, including heart disease, high cholesterol, arthritis, alcoholism, autism, hyperactivity, nervous stress, minor brain damage, neuroses of all types, and especially schizophrenia.

Well-documented evidence exists to prove niacin's positive role in treating high blood cholesterol, a well-established risk factor in coronary heart disease. In a study performed in 1955 it was found that nicotinic acid was responsible for a 22 percent reduction in cholesterol concentration in subjects with serum cholesterol levels in excess of 250 mg per 100 ml. Other studies have produced similar results. Reduction of serum triglycerides by as much as 56 percent has also been reported. The verdict seems to be that in megadoses niacin may have a slight effect in preventing the recurrence of minor heart attacks, but there is no evidence to prove it can increase a heart attack victim's chances of survival. Treatment with niacin, however, is not without its serious side effects, as we'll see when we examine its toxicity.

A clearinghouse for information on orthomolecular psychiatry (that which is based on treatment with large quantities of naturally occurring substances such as vitamins), estimates that there are currently approximately two thousand psychiatrists in the U.S. who are proponents of this approach that holds that schizophrenia and other mental disorders are diseases of deficiency or imbalance of substances in the brain. The concept first gained recognition in the '50s when similarities were noted between the symptoms of pellagra patients and schizophrenics and large doses of niacin were administered to the schizophrenics with apparent success.

Claims for the success of megavitamin treatment (which is, by the way, almost always used in conjunction with conventional treatment) abound and numerous studies have been performed, but these have yet to meet with the approval of the American Psychiatric Association (APA). After evaluation of the evidence available, the APA has concluded that megavitamin therapy is of no value. As of this writing, the use of megadoses in the treatment of mental disorders is in need of further investigation and some well-designed double-blind studies. And that will be no easy task considering the subjective nature of mental disorders, the conflicting opinions regarding the criteria for diagnosing schizophrenia, and the fact that no suitable niacin placebo has been found (niacin causes severe, visible flushing, placebos don't).

As for the other ills mentioned—alcoholism, arthritis, autism, etc.—there is currently no evidence to recommend niacin in their treatment.

TOXICITY

Megadoses of niacin are not without their dangers. First of all, it must be noted that only nicotinic acid and certain related forms, not nicotinamide, are effective in lowering cholesterol. As always seems to be the case with such things, it is also nicotinic acid that results in toxic side effects. While its effectiveness against high cholesterol levels is accepted, it is also generally agreed upon that niacin should only be used in such treatment in severe cases where altered diet and other forms of treatment alone are not effective, or where patients exhibit sensitivity to other medications. One of the more serious consequences for coronary patients of megadoses of niacin is the increased incidence of irregular heartbeat. But that's only the beginning of the story.

Minor symptoms of niacin overdose include flushing, excessive sweating, decreased appetite, abdominal pain and frequent and/or painful urination. Biochemical changes abound, including a rise in serum uric acid, which can exacerbate gout in those who are susceptible. Gastrointestinal distress is also common, with many patients developing peptic ulcers and others reporting reactivation of ulcers. Excess niacin is also implicated in liver damage and can impair carbohydrate utilization in diabetics and glucose tolerance in normal subjects. It is also important to consider this important observation by Dr. Victor Herbert: "The fact that the serum lipid level may be lower with megadoses of niacin is not necessarily desirable. It is undesirable to lower the serum lipid level if the mechanism used to lower the serum lipid level drives the lipid into tissues."

Niacin analogs that exhibit less toxicity than the free acid form are only now in the testing stages. Some of the toxic symptoms of niacin megadosing are relatively harmless and reversible, to be sure, but others are very serious indeed. The only ailment, aside from pellagra, for which niacin has been shown to be effective, is high serum cholesterol. But no one should undergo niacin treatment for this disorder except under a doctor's care so that they can be frequently monitored for heart, liver and gastrointestinal abnormalities.

RDA AND AVAILABILITY

Extensive tests have shown that an intake of 9.2 to 13.3 mg of niacin will prevent the symptoms of pellagra. The RDA for niacin has been set at a ratio of 6.6 niacin equivalents per 1000 calories; with diets of two thousand calories or less, the niacin intake still should not fall below 13 mg. That works out to a recommendation of 18 mg of niacin for men aged 23 to 50, and 13 for women.

In terms of its behavior, niacin is one of the best vitamins in the world. It's readily obtained, it's cheap (or at least many of the foods in which it abundantly occurs are), and it's quite stable in the face of light, heat, oxygen and other assailants. Cooking barely fazes it, unless it is cooked in water that is subsequently drained off.

Top-notch sources of the vitamin are lean meat, fish and poultry, but legumes, and both whole and fortified grains are also fine sources. Although the conversion of tryptophan to niacin seems miniscule at a rate of 60:1, it is really quite significant in high-protein foods. For example, a two-piece serving of chicken has 5.8 mg of preformed niacin (which is in itself pretty impressive in light of the RDA), but it also has 125 mg of tryptophan, for a total niacin content of 7.9 mg. Likewise, a cup of milk, whose niacin content looks insignificant at 0.2 mg, actually provides 2.1 mg when its tryptophan content is taken into account.

One final note about this vitamin: Although, as Kreutler notes, "niacin was first identified as a product of the oxidation of nicotine, this component of tobacco has no vitamin activity." Thus, smokers will have to look for another rationalization for continuing to light up!

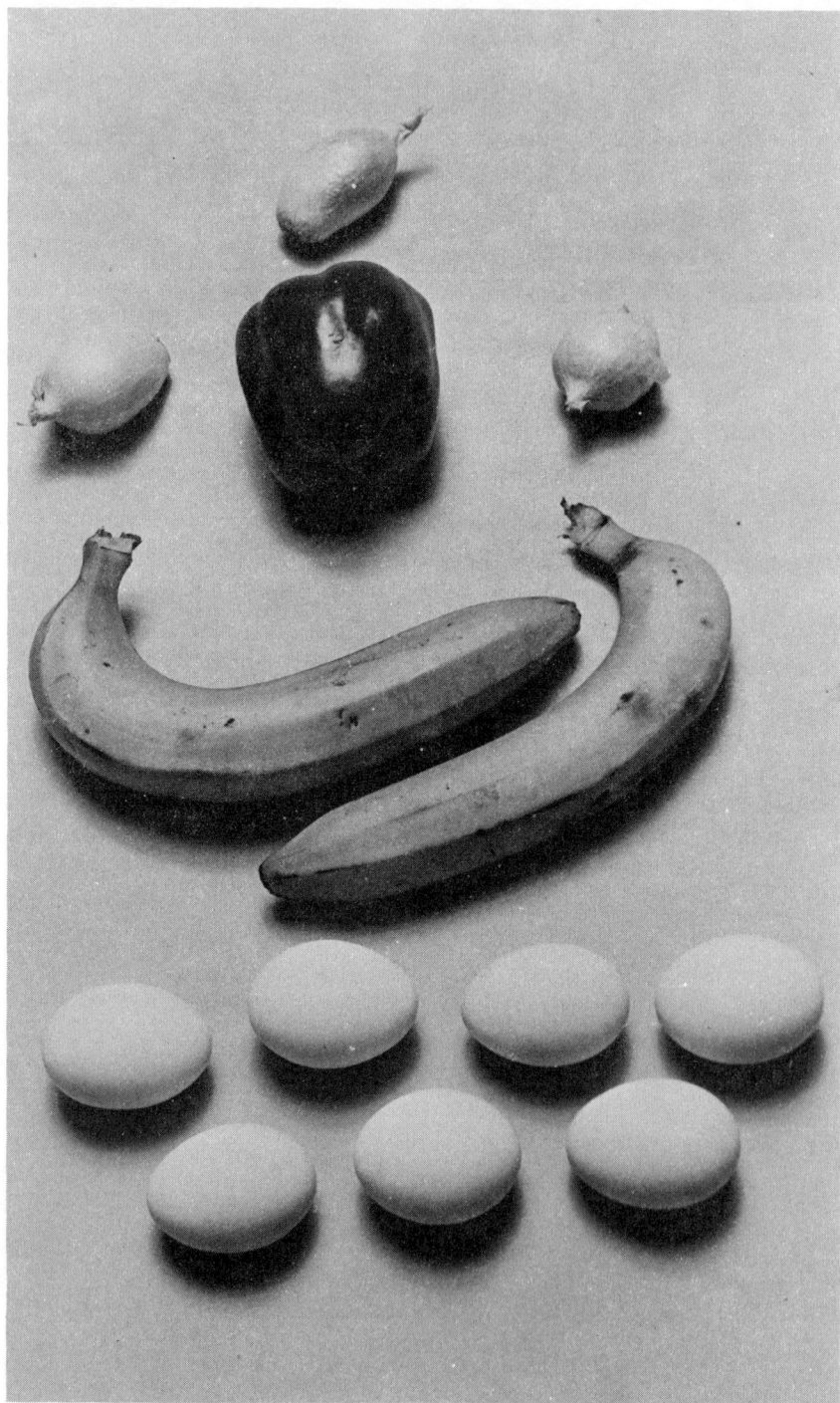

8

Vitamin B6 (Pyridoxine)

FORM AND FUNCTION

To illustrate just how closely related are the vitamins of the B-complex, Paul Gyorgy proved in 1934 what others suspected, that the B2 complex contained another chemical substance besides riboflavin. When isolated the same year, the new vitamin, pyridoxine, proved to be the elusive cure for acrodynia (dermatitis), which scientists had been seeking, when tested on rats. The vitamin was synthesized in 1939.

Vitamin B6 occurs naturally in foods in three forms: pyridoxine or pyridoxol, pyridoxal and pyridoxamine. The former occurs more readily in plant foods, while the latter two are more often found in animal foods. All three forms are equally active. "Pyridoxine" or "vitamin B6" is generally used as an umbrella term for any or all three of the forms.

Once it is absorbed in the upper portion of the small intestine, addition of phosphate to the vitamin in the body converts it to the active coenzyme form that is essential to the metabolism of protein. All three forms of pyridoxine can be converted to the coenzyme, but it is usually pyridoxal phosphate that functions in metabolic activities, although pyridoxamine phosphate also catalyzes certain reactions.

A list of B6's chores leaves no question as to its status as an essential nutrient. While B6 isn't directly involved in the production of energy, it has a vital role in the metabolism of amino acids. B6 makes itself available to a number of enzymes that synthesize and break down amino acids into their usable parts and produce harmless metabolites. B6 renders amino acids available for conversion to energy when needed and functions in converting tryptophan to niacin, producing heme, the protein base of red blood cells, converting glycogen to glucose and producing hormones, antibodies and neurotransmitters. To a lesser extent, B6 may be involved in carbohydrate and fatty acid metabolism.

Because of its long list of required activities, pyridoxine is present in all of the body's tissues, but there is no real storage of the vitamin. The unused portion of each day's supply is excreted in the urine, primarily as pyridoxic acid.

DEFICIENCY

Vitamin B6 deficiency appears to be a rarity unless artificially induced. The effects of B6 deficiency were graphically illustrated in the '50s when infants were fed a commercial formula in which the pyridoxine content was inadvertently destroyed in processing. The resulting symptoms included hyperirritability, abdominal distress, vomiting, weight loss and convulsions. In adults, pyridoxine deficiency has been experimentally induced with purified diets and the administration of an antagonist such as deoxypyridoxine. Symptoms include depression and confusion, convulsions, dermatitis, nausea and inflammation and lesions of the mouth and tongue. B6 deficiency may also result in microcytic anemia (maturation of red blood cells is inhibited so that they are smaller than normal), which is characterized by weakness, irritability, and difficulty in walking. Other effects are impaired antibody production, and rises in the xanthurenic and oxalic acid levels, the former associated with impaired glucose tolerance, the latter with the formation of kidney stones.

There is reason to suspect that the elderly population may not be getting adequate amounts of pyridoxine; deficiency is also a problem among alcoholics. The chances of B6 deficiency increase among women who are pregnant or nursing, so the RDA for these groups has been set at an additional 0.6 and 0.5 mg, respectively. Plasma levels of pyridoxal phosphate are lowered in 15 to 20 percent of women who are taking oral contraceptives, but it is as yet unclear whether such women who consume adequate diets are truly deficient in the vitamin. Altered tryptophan metabolism—caused either by B6 deficiency or estrogen interference—may be the cause of depression and impaired glucose tolerance in some users of the Pill. Women with naturally high estrogen levels may be subject to the same kind of symptoms.

Many nutritionists believe that decreases of B6 levels with oral contraceptives are neither serious nor widespread enough to warrant routine supplementation of the vitamin when the Pill is prescribed. Women who are concerned about the possibility of B6 deficiency, however, should check with the physician who writes their prescription for oral contraceptives, as certain symptoms associated with oral contraceptives can be alleviated with large doses of vitamin B6. Considering the relative lack of toxicity symptoms associated with B6 and the belief of some that oral contraceptives may cause a deficit of the vitamin that can't be compensated for with diet alone, this may be one instance in which a *little* vitamin insurance is in order.

There are a number of other drugs that can interfere with the metabolism of B6 and possibly cause deficiency with long-term use. These include chloramphenicol. INH, penicillamine, and hydralazine.

As further concerns B6 deficiency, Kreutler makes the following note: "There is increasing concern based on recent evidence that present-day normal American diets may be somewhat low in vitamin B6. Although no clinical signs have been documented, biochemical evidence of borderline 'deficiency' has been obtained in some studies. This points up the need for further study, appropriate food choices, and perhaps supplementation in some cases."

WHAT CAN IT DO?

As already noted, vitamin B6 can alleviate some of the symptoms associated with the use of oral contraceptives, *if* women on the Pill exhibit biochemical evidence of vitamin B6 deficiency. Women who consume inadequate or merely marginal diets are most at risk and should be receiving either B6 supplements or improved nutrition. The latter is preferable, for oral contraceptives affect a great many more of the body's essential substances besides B6.

B6 is also a useful treatment when various drugs or disorders interfere with the vitamin's absorption or metabolism. Conditions that can interfere with absorption, according to Kreutler, are "acute infantile celiac disease (a malabsorption syndrome), chronic alcoholism (in which synthetic preparations of the vitamin appear to be more easily absorbed), and intestinal bypass operations (sometimes used as a treatment for extreme obesity)."

Claims frequently made for B6 are prevention of morning sickness and post-operative nausea, cure of hemorrhoids and migraine headaches, and prevention and cure of kidney stones. Controlled studies and available evidence do not substantiate any of these claims. Pyridoxine does, however, seem to be an effective treatment for the carpal tunnel syndrome, a nerve condition in the hand.

TOXICITY

One group in particular that should avoid large doses of pyridoxine is sufferers of Parkinson's disease who are undergoing treatment with levodopa; B6 interferes with the action of this drug.

Otherwise, B6 seems to be without harmful effects. However, Kreutler notes slight side effects such as sleepiness with therapeutic doses up to 150 mg. Intakes of around 200 mg per day can result in B6 dependency, with symptoms such as nervousness when large doses are stopped. This same type of dependency may occur in infants whose mothers took massive doses of B6 during pregnancy; a high requirement for the vitamin can remain throughout the lifetime of such a child.

RDA AND AVAILABILITY

Because pyridoxine is so closely associated with protein metabolism, B6 requirement is based on protein intake. Based on the level of protein consumption in the U.S. (which, to the chagrin of nutritionists and the joy of supplement salesmen, usually greatly exceeds the RDA for protein), a daily dietary allowance of 2.2 mg (for males over 19) and 2.0 (for females over 19) has been set by the Food and Nutrition Board. To arrive at these figures, the Board relied on the Dietary Standard for Canada, which has suggested a ratio of 0.02 mg of B6 per gram of protein eaten.

As with the other B vitamins, top-notch sources of B6 include meat (particularly organ meats), fish and poultry, whole grains (most of the B6 content is lost in refined products), legumes, bananas, and green, leafy vegetables. B6 does not fare well in processing, so, as Marion McGill and Orrea Pye suggest in *The No-Nonsense Guide to Food & Nutrition*, "As people eat more and more precooked, preheated foods, vitamin B6 deficiency could become a clinical reality."

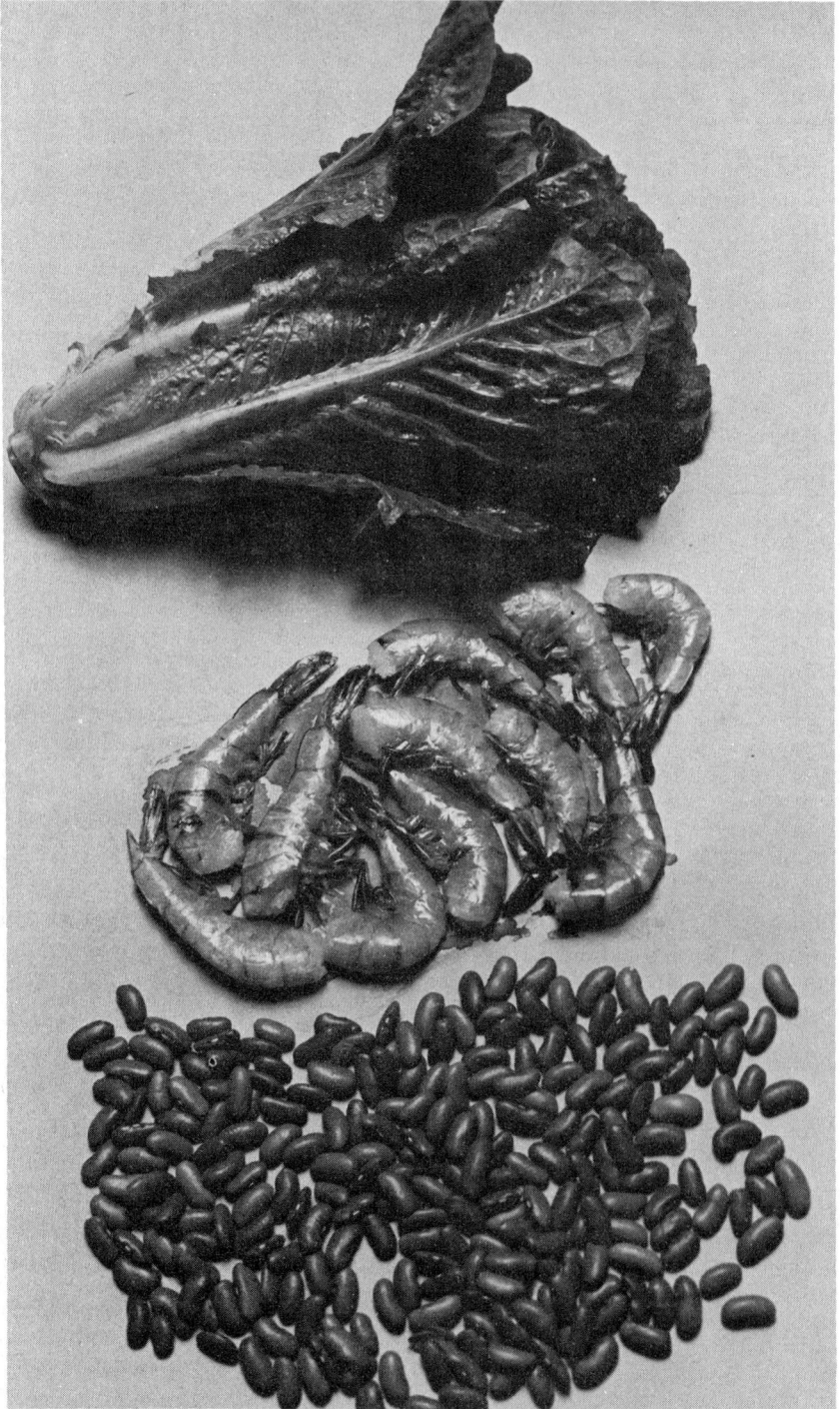

9

Folacin

FORM AND FUNCTION

When, in the early '30s, a type of anemia prevalent among pregnant women in India and capable of being induced in laboratory monkeys on a refined diet, responded to neither the known vitamins nor the liver extract found to be effective against pernicious anemia, it was time to ferret out yet another essential nutrient. Dr. Lucy Wills found yeast to contain the effective substance. It was not until 1941 that this antianemia or "Wills Factor" was isolated from spinach. Called folic acid (from the Latin *folium* or "leaf"), the new vitamin was found to be the cure for megaloblastic or macrocytic anemia (characterized by abnormally large red blood cells).

The chemical name for this vitamin is pteroylglutamic acid (PGA) for its structure of pteridine, para-aminobenzoic acid (PABA) and up to seven molecules of glutamic acid. These various forms of the vitamin vary in nutritional effectiveness, stability and availability; thus, "folate activity" is an expression sometimes used to indicate the potency of a food's entire folacin content. The term folic acid refers to the simplest or monoglutamate form of the vitamin. This and the other forms are referred to singly or collectively as folacin or folate.

Before it can be absorbed in the upper portion of the small intestine, folacin must be divested of most of its glutamate molecules. Thus, the simpler forms of the vitamin (i.e., folic acid, which is sparse in foods, but the preferred form in most supplements), are more readily absorbed. Evidence suggests that pure folic acid is absorbed almost completely by the body, while other types are

65

absorbed to lesser degrees. It appears that only 25 to 50 percent of dietary folacin may be nutritionally available.

The main task of folacin or PGA-containing coenzymes is, as the Food and Nutrition Board succinctly states it, "the transport of fragments containing a single carbon atom from one compound to another." If that sounds like a menial task, think for a moment about its implications. Folacin's action is necessary for amino acid metabolism and the synthesis of all nucleotides, one of the most important of which is thymine, an essential ingredient of deoxyribonucleic acid, better known as DNA. As we know, DNA carries the genes that are blueprints for new cells. Without DNA, cells do not divide and organisms do not grow. Thus, as Kreutler says, the absence of folacin from the diet "interferes with DNA synthesis and therefore cell division, resulting in enlarged but undivided red blood cell precursors." As a component of DNA, folacin is necessary to every cell in the body, but its absence is particularly crucial to those (i.e., red blood cells, cells lining the intestinal tract, etc.) that are being replaced on a daily basis.

DEFICIENCY

Macrocytic or megaloblastic anemia is, of course, the major deficiency disease associated with folacin. However, based on its role in DNA synthesis, it can affect every cell of the body. Thus, a shortage of folacin in youngsters can result in stunted growth. Folacin deficiency can wreak havoc with the intestinal tract, where cell turnover is rapid. Among the damage is an impaired ability to absorb nutrients from food. A swollen, inflamed tongue is another symptom of folacin deficiency. The body's ability to fight infection may also be impaired, as folacin is also necessary to white blood cell production.

The human body is most susceptible to folacin deficiency in times of growth, when cell division—and hence DNA synthesis—progresses at a rapid rate. Thus, onset of deficiency symptoms is more rapid—and common—among pregnant and nursing women, infants and children. The hormonal changes of pregnancy also account for increased need.

As with B6 and some of the other water-soluble vitamins, women taking oral contraceptives have lower blood levels of folacin. In a report on the use of oral contraceptives, Dr. David P. Rose notes that eighty cases of macrocytic anemia were reported between 1968 and 1977 among women on the Pill. Still, disagreement is rampant among researchers as to the seriousness of the reduced blood levels of this vitamin. Indeed, in half the studies undertaken, reduced blood levels were not shown to exist. Differing results may reflect different nutritional states of the subjects. Dr. Janet C. King offers another interesting perspective on the problem:

"The lack of agreement among studies on the effect of OCA's (oral contraceptive agents) on vitamin metabolism suggests that the individual response to steroid treatment is varied. Some women may be more sensitive to the effects of OCA's than others. This is particularly evident for folacin and vitamin B6 metabolism. About twenty percent of the OCA users who were tested had enlarged cervical and vaginal cells probably indicative of abnormal folacin metabolism. In all cases oral folacin supplementation corrected the abnormality. These women should probably receive supplements of about 100 mcg folacin while using contraceptive steroids."

Other drugs interfere with folacin, as well. Among these Kreutler identifies aminosalicylic acid and cycloserine (used in the treatment of tuberculosis), and some anticonvulsants, which interfere with absorption, and trimethoprim and pyrimethamine (used in the treatment of malaria), which inactivate folacin. A cancer chemotherapy drug called methotrexate also inactivates the vitamin, but in this case the action is deliberate. We know how important cell division is to the growth of cancers and how important folacin is to cell division. Thus, methotrexate was synthesized to masquerade as folic acid and prevent the cell from properly using the vitamin. Because cells cannot function without folacin, they die. The only trouble with such medications (this one is being used primarily in the treatment of leukemia and breast and bone cancers) is that they don't limit their activities to cancerous cells.

As with everything else, alcoholics are likely to find themselves in short supply of folacin. Kreutler, in fact, contends that chronic alcoholics lose their ability to absorb dietary forms of the vitamin and should be receiving synthetic supplements. According to Brody, "Persons with chronic infections, cancer, or chronic loss of red blood cells require additional folacin."

WHAT CAN IT DO?

Folacin can be used in the treatment of macrocytic anemia *if* the possibility of B12 deficiency has been completely ruled out (See "Toxicity" next page). Patients with certain diseases—arthritis, atherosclerosis, some psychological disorders, etc.—have shown lowered levels of folacin, but there is no evidence to suggest that folacin deficiency is the cause of such diseases or that folacin supplementation is the cure. As you're no doubt probably tired of hearing, this is yet another avenue along which further investigation needs to be directed.

TOXICITY

Folacin can cure the symptoms of megaloblastic anemia, which can also be caused by a shortage of vitamin B12. It cannot, however, cure the much more serious condition of pernicious anemia, an inherent disease that prevents B12 absorption, but may effectively mask the disease so that it goes undiagnosed. Untreated, pernicious anemia results in irreversible brain damage and eventually death. Allowing pernicious anemia to go undiagnosed is probably, therefore, the greatest danger of self-prescribed folacin supplementation. Otherwise, doses of as much as 400 mg a day for five months or 10 mg a day for five years have shown no effects in adults.

RDA AND AVAILABILITY

A lot of unanswered questions about folacin make it difficult to determine both the real, usable folacin content of foods and the precise amount required by the body. As already noted, it is believed that only about 25 to 50 percent of dietary folacin is nutritionally available. Evidence also suggests that 100 to 220 mcg of the vitamin is needed daily to maintain tissue reserves. Based on these assumptions, the RDA for men and women has been set at 400 mcg. Because of increased DNA synthesis and cell division, RDAs for pregnant and lactating women are considerably higher at 800 mcg for the former and 500 mcg for the latter.

As its name suggests, folacin is abundant in green, leafy vegetables. Legumes are a good source, as are fish, liver and most other meats.

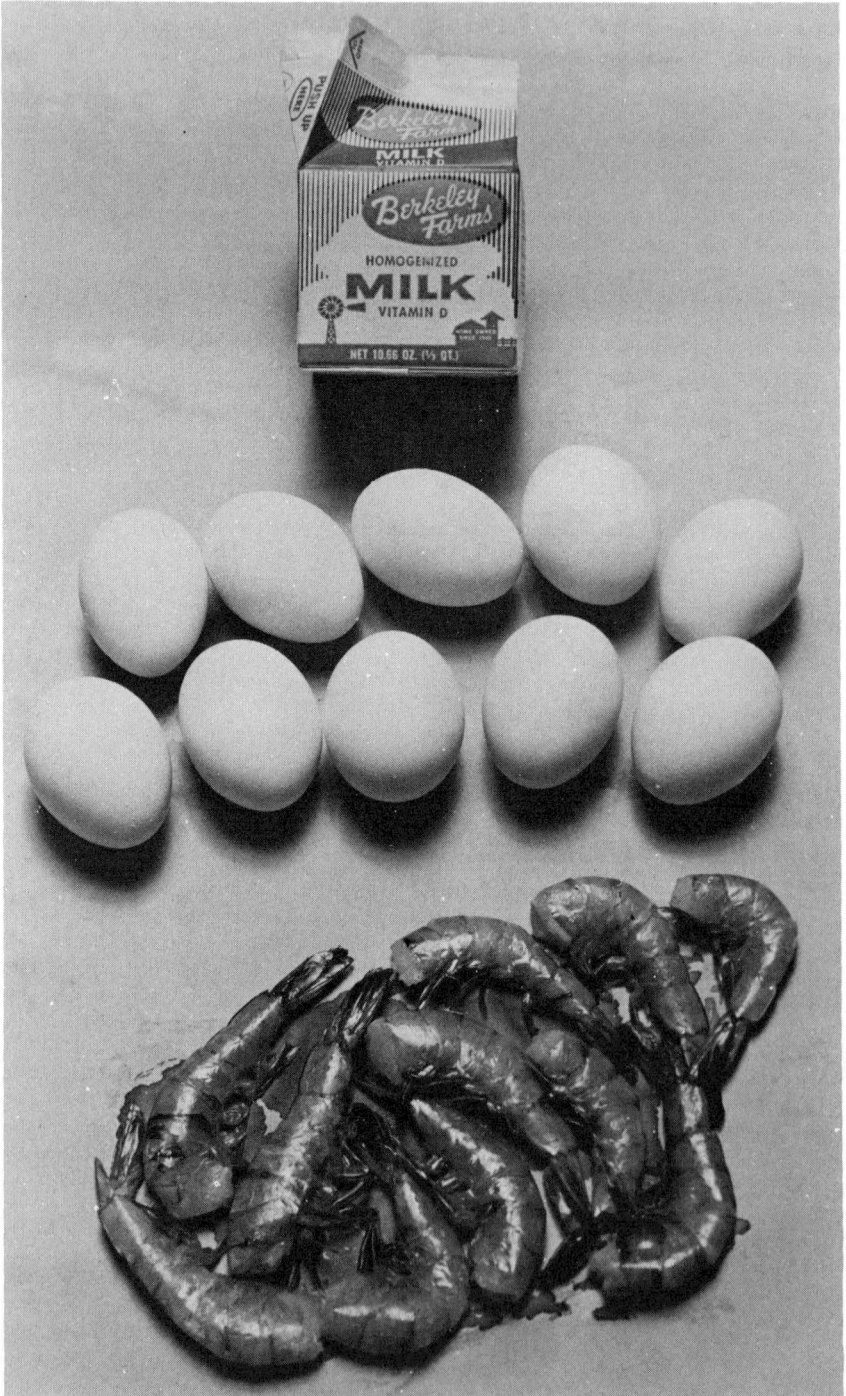

10

Vitamin B12 (Cobalamin)

FORM AND FUNCTION

With the discovery of the last of the B vitamins came the power to deal with yet another deadly deficiency disease. "Pernicious," says Webster's dictionary, "applies to that which does great harm by insidiously undermining or weakening." When teamed with "anemia," "pernicious" means slow, but inevitable death. The first clue to this ruthless riddle came in 1926 with the unlikely discovery that a pound of raw liver a day could cure the symptoms of pernicious anemia, a disease characterized by a reduced number of red blood cells, weakness, gastrointestinal and neurological disturbances, etc. After that, the slow but steady hunt for the responsible food factor was on.

Intrigued by the fact that so much liver was necessary for successful treatment, and aware that pernicious anemia sufferers had unusual gastric secretions, William Castle theorized that an intrinsic factor produced by the body was necessary to team with the extrinsic factor to be found in foods such as liver. Sufferers of pernicious anemia, went his theory, probably lacked the means to produce this important intrinsic factor.

Thanks to Castle's theory and a common microorganism that also needed the as-yet-unidentified vitamin for its survival, vitamin B12 was isolated in 1948 by two teams of researchers working independently. According to *The Vitamin Book*, one ton of liver was required to produce 20 mg of the vitamin. Vitamin B12 was finally synthesized in 1973.

The three most common forms of B12 found in animal foods—and in human blood and tissues—are methylcobalamin, adenosylcobalamin, and hydroxycobalamin. A fourth type, cyanocobalamin,

71

is less commonly found in the diet, but is the most stable form and the one produced for commercial supplements. Cobalamin is often used as a generic term for vitamin B12, but is not entirely appropriate as there are a number of cobalamins that are nutritionally inactive. Likewise, another general descriptive term used for the vitamin—cyanocobalamin—is no more appropriate as it refers only to a single form of the vitamin.

Perhaps B12 eluded researchers so long because it is such an oddball of a vitamin. First of all, it must have both intrinsic factor (sometimes called Castle's intrinsic factor or IF) and calcium in order to carry out its duties. Next, it is the only vitamin that has an inorganic element—cobalt—as part of its complex structure. Finally, it can be synthesized *only* by bacteria. Plants do not make it and it can be produced in animals only by microorganisms in the intestinal tract. For most animals this is apparently a good source of the vitamin (hence the inability to find suitable test animals for B12 research), while in man the vitamin is thought to be synthesized too far down the intestinal tract to be absorbed.

Absorption of *dietary* B12 occurs much farther up the gastrointestinal tract, in the ileum, the lower part of the small intestine where it opens into the large intestine. But, as we know, it needs a bit of help to get there. B12 enters the body in the company of cobalamin-binding proteins found in food, milk, etc., but these guys don't seem to meet its needs and are rubbed out by protein-digesting enzymes from the pancreas. B12 then takes up with the intrinsic factor, which is a large glycoprotein secreted by the stomach. The IF effortlessly guides B12 to receptor sites on the ileum, which are the only places the vitamin can be absorbed, and attaches itself there until the vitamin is taken in. Absorption may also occur by simple diffusion, a process Kreutler describes as, "The passive movement of substances from an area of high concentration to one of low concentration. Water and certain water-soluble nutrient molecules enter the cells of the intestinal lining via diffusion." This process, however, probably accounts for the absorption of only about 1 to 3 percent of B12. However, when megadoses—or enough raw liver—are administered, this type of absorption bebomes significant.

Once absorbed (the smaller the dose of B12 the more efficient is the IF transport system), B12 bids farewell to its old friend IF and continues its journey through the general circulation under the care of transcobalamin II, a transport protein. In terms of bodily need, the liver stores much more B12 than other water-soluble vitamins and has an efficient recycling system for the vitamin that precludes its daily intake.

There are a number of good reasons why the body goes to so much trouble to get B12 and hangs onto it so tenaciously once it's got it. Small as our requirement for this vitamin is, it is involved in the metabolism and utilization of all of the basic nutrients and has key functions in every cell of the body. First of all, B12 is needed along with folacin for DNA synthesis. As pointed out in the chapter on folacin, this genetic material is most urgently needed by cells that are constantly replenished, and is therefore critical to the formation of red blood cells. Thus, a deficiency of either folacin or B12 can result in megaloblastic anemia.

Pernicious anemia (the inability to produce intrinsic factor and thus absorb B12) is so devastating to the nervous system because of B12's important role in the formation and feeding of nerve cells. It is not only involved in the metabolism of carbohydrates needed to fuel nerve cells, but is a component of the material (myelin) that forms the protective sheath around them.

DEFICIENCY

A deficiency of vitamin B12 or folacin results in megaloblastic anemia, but in the case of B12 deficiency, the enlarged but undivided blood cells and gastrointestinal trouble are accompanied by damage to the nervous system. Pernicious anemia, as already noted, is caused not by a shortage of B12 in the diet, but by the inability of the body to produce the intrinsic factor that makes it absorbable. Pernicious anemia is probably an inherited disorder that often shows up late in life.

The body requires such small amounts of B12, and recycles it so efficiently, that dietary deficiency is rare. It does occur among vegans, vegetarians who consume no animal products, but lacto-ovo vegetarians (those who consume milk and eggs) get enough of the vitamin. B12 deficiency is a particular problem among children who are fed strict vegetarian diets and nursing infants of mothers who are vegans. Because they have no B12 stores in the liver, anemia shows rapid onset among such children.

Adults, on the other hand, who adopt vegan diets later in life, may not exhibit deficiency symptoms for some time, often about five to six years. Some do not develop deficiency symptoms at all. It has been suggested that, over time, they may adjust to trace amounts that may be found in some plant foods due to fermentation or the bacterial content of soil and water. For infants and children, however, the problem is much more serious and immediate. As Kreutler suggests, pregnant and lactating women, infants and children should have, if not meat, at least milk and/or eggs in the diet. Otherwise, B12 supplementation is a necessity.

Women on oral contraceptives may have lowered B12 levels, as may those who use the diabetes drugs metformin and phenformin. Further, Dr. Victor Herbert and his colleagues have presented evidence that large doses of vitamin C can destroy substantial amounts of vitamin B12. Others have challenged their findings. Persons who undergo surgical removal of the ileum or a portion of the stomach are subject to vitamin B12 deficiencies, as well. In such cases, as with adult vegans, symptoms do not ordinarily occur for about five years or so, when liver stores are depleted.

WHAT CAN IT DO?

Oral supplements of vitamin B12 can be used to treat dietary deficiencies, which are rare here except among vegans. In fact, oral supplementation is highly recommended for followers of such diets. However, individuals with pernicious anemia, absorptive disorders or those who have undergone surgical removal of the stomach or ileum, should be under a doctor's care and receiving B12 injections. On the other hand, these injections, which seem to be a favorite placebo among doctors and patients alike, are, like oral megadoses, of no benefit in the absence of a true B12 deficiency. In short, if you are getting an adequate supply of B12 (which is an incredibly small amount and one easily obtained in normal diets), more of the vitamin will be of no value. Contrary to claims, additional B12 does not pep you up, cure depression or other mental disorders, build better blood, or wipe out that advertising agency invention: "tired blood." Vitamin B12 has proved an effective treatment for cyanide poisoning, particularly in the hydroxycobalamin form, which could be a useful application for those who think laetrile is a harmless substance.

TOXICITY

While large amounts of B12 over long periods do not seem to produce any adverse effects, they, like megadoses of folacin, can be harmful to individuals with pernicious anemia who are treating themselves by guesswork with oral doses rather than seeing a physician for diagnosis and proper treatment.

RDA AND AVAILABILITY

Storage and lifespan of vitamin B12 are such that it is not necessary to consume the vitamin on a daily basis. Based on estimated body pool size and turnover time for the vitamin, plus a large built-in margin of safety, the Food and Nutrition Board has set the RDA for most adults at 3.0 mcg. Pregnant women and those who are nursing are thought to need an extra microgram. The average American diet contains between 5 and 15 mcg, though individual diets range from as low as 1 mcg to as high as 100 mcg. Those consuming ordinary diets should have no trouble at all, particularly if meals include meat (especially liver, which provides over twenty-two times the RDA in a single three-ounce serving), fish, milk and eggs. Kreutler recommends 15 mcg per day "for those whose liver stores are depleted by illness (fever or hyperthyroidism, for example)."

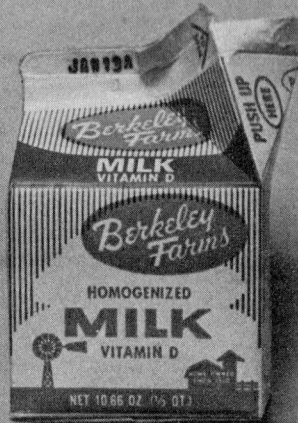

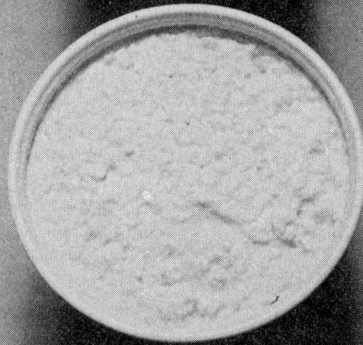

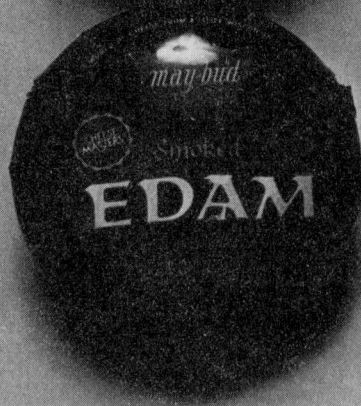

11

Biotin

FORM AND FUNCTION

So potent is the B vitamin biotin that its requirement is in micrograms, prompting some to call it a "micromicronutrient." In terms of its discovery, it seems that during the early part of this century, all roads led to biotin. It was probably "discovered" more than any other vitamin and had at least six names, including vitamin H and protective factor X. As with riboflavin, somewhere in the course of its discovery, someone noticed that biotin possessed a remarkable similarity to a growth-stimulating substance called coenzyme R. Other researchers, including Margaret Boas, observed that rats fed a diet of uncooked egg whites developed symptoms such as dermatitis, weight and hair loss, paralysis, and hemorrhaging under the skin, which could be reversed by cooking the egg whites or by adding other foods to the diet.

The vitamin was isolated from the yolks of duck eggs in 1936 and called biotin by Fritz Kogl. Paul Gyorgy proved that biotin, some other independently discovered substances and his own vitamin H were the very same thing. Biotin became officially recognized as a vitamin in 1943 after its chemical structure was identified and it was synthesized in the laboratory.

Functioning as a coenzyme, biotin certainly pulls its own weight in the body, participating in a whole handful of metabolic reactions. Biotin is known to function in fatty acid synthesis and amino acid metabolism. Kreutler notes that it may also be involved in protein and carbohydrate metabolism, antibody formation and synthesis of pancreatic amylase, an enzyme that helps convert starch to sugar.

77

One of the more interesting aspects of biotin is its synthesis by bacteria in the intestinal tract. There is reason to believe that this home-grown version of the vitamin is absorbed and used by the body; it may even provide a goodly portion of the body's requirement. One reason to think so is that the body excretes more biotin in the urine and feces than it takes in in the diet. Most biotin storage takes place in the liver and kidneys, though the vitamin is found in all cells of the body. Storage consists of only minute amounts.

DEFICIENCY

Biotin occurs so abundantly in foods and is needed in such tiny amounts that a natural deficiency in humans is not known to exist. Deficiency can be artificially induced in humans and animals on a diet of raw egg whites. Symptoms are similar to those of the rats mentioned earlier and include drying and discoloration of the skin, loss of hair and appetite, muscle pain, and lethargy. Raw egg white, it turns out, contains a compound called avidin that binds biotin and makes it unavailable for absorption. Avidin is certainly no threat to the average person's biotin supply, however, as it is easily destroyed in cooking. There just aren't that many people who go around eating raw eggs, and those who do would have to consume about a dozen and a half a day for a number of weeks in order to create a deficiency.

Because we apparently get much of our biotin from bacterial action in the intestinal tract, prolonged use of antibiotics could result in a secondary deficiency of the vitamin.

WHAT CAN IT DO?

Biotin is often included in vitamin megadoses and some vitamin promoters have even made claims for its powers in preventing heart disease and mental illness. There is no evidence to support such claims nor, as has been stated, is there any reason to think that *anybody* other than the very rare individual suffers from biotin deficiency.

There is evidence, however, that biotin may be a useful treatment against seborrheic dermatitis and Leiner's disease, an oily rash that sometimes afflicts infants. There is, in fact, some speculation that these may, indeed, be biotin deficiency diseases. But, while the vitamin has been shown to be effective in some cases in reversing the symptoms of these diseases in infants, it appears to have no effect on them in adults.

TOXICITY

Biotin toxicity? It doesn't seem to exist. But then, there are a lot of other things about this vitamin we don't know yet, either.

RDA AND AVAILABILITY

Nobody, not even those distinguished members of the Food and Nutrition Board who formulate the RDAs, knows how much biotin the average human needs to take in. The reason is that we are unsure how much the body makes and how much of what it makes it absorbs. As already mentioned, the combination of biotin excreted in the urine and feces exceeds that consumed in the diet. It is assumed by the Food and Nutrition Board that biotin excreted in the feces is that produced in the body, while biotin excreted in the urine is that from dietary intake. Studies show that humans excrete somewhere between 18 and 46 mcg of biotin per day in the urine. Assuming that half of dietary biotin is absorbed and excreted in the urine, approximately 100 mcg of biotin would provide replacement at the upper level of excretion. Mixed American diets provide between 100 and 300 mcg of biotin per day. While there is no RDA for biotin, there is now an "estimated safe and adequate daily dietary intake" of 100 to 200 mcg for adults. Figures are considerably lower for infants and children.

At 100 to 300 mcg per day in the diet, Americans are getting far more biotin than their counterparts in Western Europe who consume only about 50 to 100 mcg per day. If they aren't experiencing deficiencies, there is no reason to think we should. Biotin occurs in a wide variety of foods, with particularly good sources including liver, kidney, egg yolk and some vegetables. Milk and other dairy products are also good sources in the American diet. It is also important to note that the biotin in some foods—notably wheat— is chemically bound in such a way as to make it unavailable to test animals and, theoretically, to humans. The biotin content of many foods has not yet been determined.

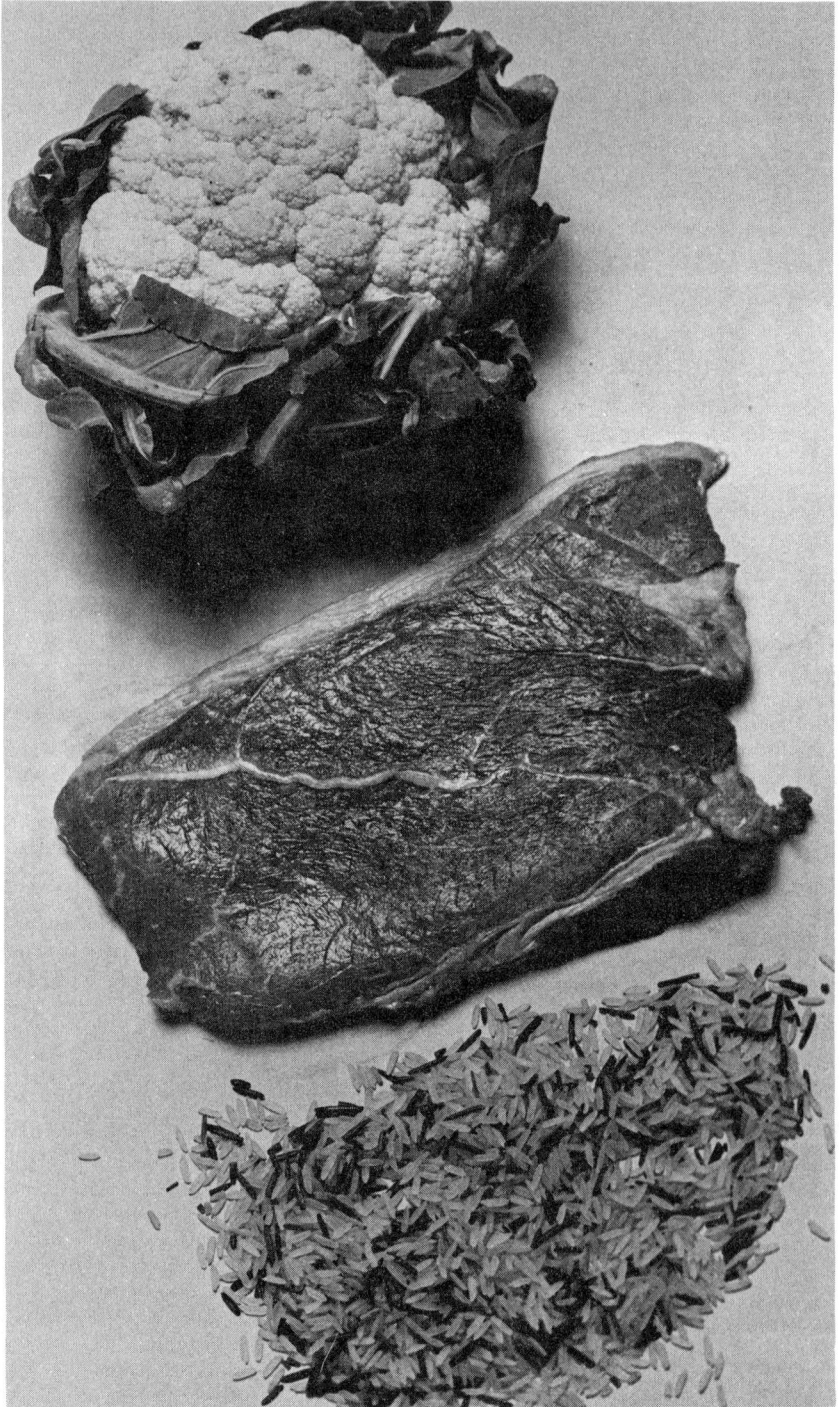

12

Pantothenic Acid

FORM AND FUNCTION

The first "discovery" of biotin in 1901 was actually the discovery of a substance called "Bios," which promoted growth in microorganisms. The complex of B vitamins to which this substance belonged, contained not only biotin, but pantothenic acid, as well. It was not until the 1930s, however, that scientists isolated the substance and found that withholding it from the diets of laboratory animals resulted in a wide array of symptoms. Between 1938 and 1940, Roger J. Williams isolated and synthesized the growth-promoting vitamin, which he called pantothenic acid from the Greek *pantos* for "everywhere." The name is an apt one, as pantothenic acid appears in all plant and animal foods. It is, as its discoverer has said, "an essential constituent of every kind of living cell."

Pantothenic acid works its myriad magic in the body as a component of both coenzyme A, responsible for some of the key chemical reactions in the body, and of acyl-carrier protein (ACP), the vehicle that carries CoA to the cells, where it is involved in the synthesis of fatty acids. CoA further functions in the all-important process of releasing energy from carbohydrates, fats and proteins, and plays a role in the synthesis of sterols (cholesterol is one of these and is important in the formation of steroid hormones; i.e., cortisone, the sex hormones, etc.), poryphyrin (the pigment component of hemoglobin) and acetylcholine (a neurotransmitter).

The body stores very limited amounts of pantothenic acid, primarily in the major organs. Further, the vitamin is thought to be

81

synthesized by bacteria in the intestines. However, we know neither the quantity nor the availability of pantothenic acid from this source.

DEFICIENCY

In humans, pantothenic acid deficiency appears to exist only where it is artificially induced for experimental purposes through the administration of a purified diet for long periods and the addition of a metabolic antagonist to the vitamin, omega-methylpantothenic acid. With an experimental diet virtually bereft of pantothenic acid, symptoms of deficiency do not begin to appear for about two-and-a-half months. Test subjects developed such symptoms as insomnia, leg cramps, numbness and tingling in the hands and feet, gastrointestinal problems, depression and irritability. They were also prone to reduced antibody production.

Induced deficiency in test animals produces a different set of symptoms in each kind of animal, but predominant among them are aborted or deformed fetuses, retarded growth, neuromuscular disorders, gastrointestinal malfunction, adrenal cortical failure, etc. There are also abnormal changes to skin, hair and feathers. Pantothenic acid-deficient rats, for example, develop gray hair.

A deficiency of pantothenic acid is very unlikely to develop alone, but may occur with other B-vitamin deficiencies in persons who are severely malnourished or do not get a wide variety of healthy foods. Kreutler notes that, "Because food processing can result in vitamin losses and because clinicians generally are not looking for pantothenic acid deficiency, concern has recently arisen that 'borderline' deficiencies may occur in people who do not consume diversified diets. More study is needed."

WHAT CAN IT DO?

If you're one of those people who feels gray hair makes you look old rather than sophisticated or distinguished, you'd probably do better to spend your money in a beauty shop rather than on large supplements of pantothenic acid. Contrary to claims—and to what happens in rates—no evidence exists to suggest that pantothenic acid will prevent or reverse the graying of hair in humans.

Despite other claims—including some by Williams, the vitamin's discoverer—and some interesting results in test animals, there is no scientific proof that widespread pantothenic acid deficiency is responsible for miscarriage, birth defects, arthritis, allergies, mental deficiency and mental illness, or Addison's disease (an affliction of the adrenal glands). Indeed, uninduced deficiency of the disease has not even been shown to exist. As with most of the vitamins, pantothenic acid is in need of carefully controlled studies with human beings. Kreutler observes that pantothenic acid has been used with some success to treat the neurologic symptoms of those who have received streptomycin, as well as to stimulate the gastrointestinal tract after surgery.

TOXICITY

Megadoses of pantothenic acid do not appear to be harmful to men or animals. The men in one study ingested 10 g of calcium pantothenate (the calcium salt of pantothenic acid) without incident. In a 1954 test utilizing doses of 10 to 20 grams, there were some symptoms of diarrhea and water retention.

RDA AND AVAILABILITY

The Food and Nutrition Board has not set an RDA for pantothenic acid, because there is a lack of solid evidence on which to determine dietary need. They have, however, set an "estimated safe and adequate daily intake" of 4 to 7 mg for adults; estimated adequate intakes have also been set for other age groups, based upon proportional energy needs. Diets in the U.S. have a pantothenic content that ranges from 5 to 20 mg; approximately 7 mg per day is a customary intake. The "safe and adequate" figure of 4 to 7 mg was set based on this information, urinary excretion levels and other evidence.

How can you assure that you get pantothenic acid in the diet? Don't forget the source of this vitamin's name; it literally occurs everywhere, in all foods. Like other vitamins, however, it does not occur in all foods in equal amounts. Especially rich in the vitamin are meat (particularly organ meats), legumes and whole grains. The vitamin is relatively stable in ordinary preparation, but heat above the boiling point is a serious threat to it. Likewise, freezing significantly affects the pantothenic acid levels of meats and vegetables. Wheat loses about half of its pantothenic acid in refining and it is not added back; similarly, refined rice can contain as little as one-fourth its original pantothenic acid content. Yeast, salmon, vegetables, milk and eggs are also good dietary sources.

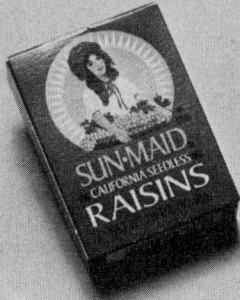

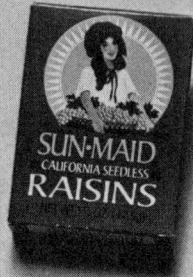

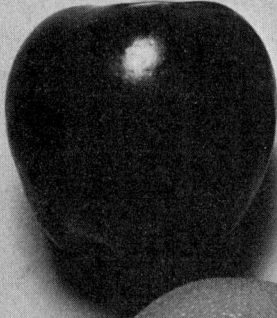

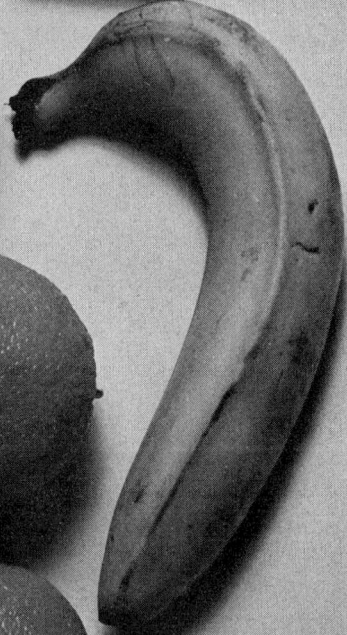

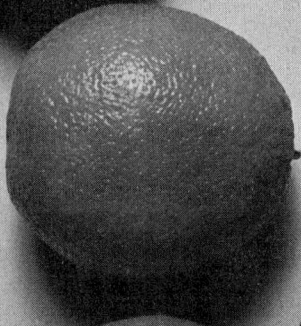

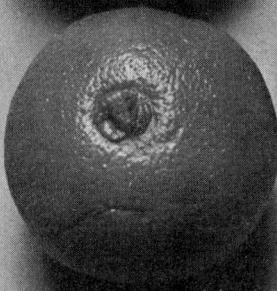

13

Vitamin C (Ascorbic Acid)

FORM AND FUNCTION

Every school child who doesn't already know it, soon learns the story of how, in 1747, a physician named James Lind used oranges and lemons to cure British sailors of scurvy. Some may even know the less familiar tale of the French explorer Jacques Cartier, who was rapidly losing his men to the disease in the winter of 1535 along the frozen St. Lawrence River. Cartier was lucky enough to receive the aid of the local Indians, who generously volunteered the cure: an extract produced from the needles and bark of pine trees.

Although, by the nature of his experiment (he added different substances to the regular diets of six different groups of men with scurvy and only those who received the oranges and lemons were cured), Lind proved rather conclusively that citrus fruit contained an anti-scurvy factor, it took the British Navy another 50 years to add lemon juice to its sailors' diets.

It was not until about 110 years later that two researchers, Axel Holst and Theodor Frohlich, managed to induce scurvy in guinea pigs with a refined diet while studying cell respiration. Then, in 1928, Albert Szent-Gyorgyi isolated from adrenal glands, then from cabbage and orange juice, a substance he believed to be hexuronic acid. C.G. King and W.A. Waugh of the University of Pittsburgh isolated the vitamin from lemon juice in 1932. It was called ascorbic acid for its antiscorbutic (anti-scurvy) properties.

There are two recognized forms of vitamin C: ascorbic acid and dehydroascorbic acid. The latter is the oxidation product of the former and has about 80 percent of its activity. Most animals, with the exception of man, the primates, guinea pigs and a few other species, are able to synthesize their own ascorbic acid from sugars and do not need it in the diet.

In humans, vitamin C enters the body through the small intestine and is carried via the portal vein to the liver from whence it is distributed throughout the body. Although the symptoms of scurvy do not begin to appear until the body's store of the vitamin falls below 300 mg, the human body maintains a reserve of approximately 1500 mg of the vitamin. Most of it is found in the liver, spleen and adrenal glands. About three percent of this reserve is excreted every day. Animals that synthesize their own ascorbic acid are thought to maintain their tissues at the saturation level or maximum concentration. Though it is not the point of view of the Food and Nutrition Board, which sees no advantage to the practice, some scientists feel that it should be the goal of humans to maintain their tissues at the saturation level, as well. In the average adult that state would amount to approximately 4000 milligrams of the vitamin. At the three-percent-a-day depletion rate, it would require an intake of about 120 mg per day to maintain saturation. At the present time, however, the RDA for adults is 60 mg, although in the past it has been set at both 45 and 75 mg.

Once the saturation level of vitamin C is reached, its excretion rate rises markedly. When 100 mg or less of the vitamin is ingested, daily absorption efficiency is approximately 80 to 90 percent. Efficiency drops at higher intakes.

Vitamin C has been assigned a number of important tasks in the body. At the top of its list is its role in the formation of collagen, the protein component of every square millimeter of the connective tissue that holds the body's cells (and the body) together. It is the breakdown of this connective tissue that results in the gruesome symptoms of scurvy. One of the more immediate aspects of this job is maintaining the integrity of the blood vessels, including the capillaries; hence the fragile, easily ruptured capillaries and diffuse tissue bleeding of scurvy. Collagen is required, too, in the very important task of wound healing.

Vitamin C also participates in amino acid metabolism and the synthesis of some hormones and neurotransmitters. Other functions include combating infection, facilitating iron absorption, and protecting the essential fatty acids and vitamins A and E from oxidation.

DEFICIENCY

Once the scourge of the high seas and a major killer, first recorded as far back as 1500 B.C. in Egypt, scurvy is the disease that results from a deficiency of vitamin C. Considering the vital role of collagen in the body—and vitamin C's key role in its formation—it is little wonder that a lack of the vitamin results in such a devastating disease.

In its early stages vitamin C deficiency may result in easy bruising and bleeding gums. But with the onset of scurvy comes dry, rough, scaly, discolored skin, and hemorrhaging of the gums, on the surface of the skin, under the skin, in the muscles, and into the joints, with resultant joint pain. In addition to the bleeding, gums become spongy and swollen, with the result that teeth may loosen and fall out. Wounds do not heal properly or, if healed, may easily break open again. Anemia is another manifestation of the disease. According to Dr. Sue Rodwell Williams, "It is partially caused by hemorrhagic blood loss, but also by the faulty metabolic interrelationships of vitamin C with folic acid and iron. Concurrent deficiency of other nutrients also contributes to the anemia." Adults may also experience such symptoms as weakness, weariness and irritability.

Because of the associated joint pain, infants with scurvy often lie in the only position that's comfortable: on their backs with their knees flexed and their hips rotated outward; some have described it as a frog's leg position. They also develop extreme sensitivity, irritability and loss of appetite. As with any vitamin, a deficiency of C is particularly harmful during the growing years. Children may develop malformed bones with microscopic cracks and other growth defects.

Scurvy is rare in the U.S., but can occur in specialized cases. For instance, infants who are fed cows' milk and are not receiving supplements may be susceptible. Breast-fed babies usually do all right with the vitamin unless the mother is deficient. Ordinarily the disease does not appear for about nine months, since infants are born with a supply of the vitamin that is adequate for several months.

Cases of scurvy have been reported among individuals on bizarre, monotonous diets. Those who may have reduced levels of the vitamin are the elderly, whose diets are often less than adequate, alcoholics, heavy smokers (who can have as much as 20 to 40 percent less vitamin C in their blood than non-smokers), women on the Pill, the poor and/or nutritionally uneducated who get few fresh fruits and vegetables, some fad dieters and users of certain drugs (antibiotics, sulfa drugs, adrenal steroids, salicylates, etc.). Particularly susceptible to reduced levels are those receiving large doses of aspirin for the treatment of rheumatoid arthritis. According to Dr. Fredrick J. Stare, Chairman of the Department of Nutrition at Harvard, "Dietary surveys indicate that C is the vitamin most often found in less-than-recommended amounts in diets of all age groups." Usually the lowered level still falls within the normal range and is one that can be easily made up with a slight modification (say the addition of a glass of orange juice to the diet).

WHAT CAN IT DO?

Asking what vitamin C can do is tantamount to opening the world's biggest can of worms. There is no doubt that this vitamin is controversial....with a capital C. Most of the controversy was generated in 1970 when the Nobel Prize-winning physicist Linus Pauling published *Vitamin C and the Common Cold*. There hasn't been a peaceful moment in scientific circles ever since.

The major thrust of Pauling's book is that megadoses of C can result in 45 percent fewer colds and 60 percent fewer sick days. His prescription to acheive this goal is one to three grams (1000 to 3000 milligrams) of vitamin C per day as a preventative measure, and up to 10 grams per day when a cold has set in. Since publication of *Vitamin C And The Common Cold*, a number of interesting double-blind studies have been performed to test Pauling's hypothesis. One of these was undertaken by Dr. Terence W. Anderson and his colleagues at the University of Toronto, using 818 adult volunteers in a 14-week trial. Divided at random, half the subjects were directed to take a regular dose of one gram of ascorbic acid a day and to increase the dose to four grams during the first three days of any illness. The other group was given a placebo, an inactive substance that was identical to the ascorbic acid in appearance, taste and smell. Neither the subjects nor the investigators knew who belonged to which group.

What Anderson found was that the total number of episodes of illness was 7 percent lower in the ascorbic acid group, and that that group also had 12 percent fewer days of recorded symptoms. The researchers judged these findings to be statistically "not significant." They did, however, find a significant difference in the amount of disability experienced by the two groups. According to Anderson, "The vitamin group had recorded 531 days 'confined to the house,' some 30 percent fewer than the 769 days recorded by the placebo group. The probability of this being due to chance was less than 1 in 1000."

Subsequent trials by Anderson's group produced similar results and also showed little difference in the effect of prophylactic doses of 250, 1000 and 2000 mgm. Thus, the megadoses suggested by Pauling, Passwater and others appear to be unnecessary to achieve the limited effect C seems to have on cold symptoms; smaller doses, which easily maintain tissue saturation anyway, appear to perform just as well.

While it has been hypothesized that megadoses of vitamin C may have an antihistamine effect upon colds, Anderson concludes "that the extra vitamin C is not protecting against viruses directly, or just helping to dry up nasal secretions, but rather is helping the victim to overcome the general feeling of 'malaise' that often accompanies an acute infection, and is probably part of a non-specific reaction to stress." Anderson further suggests that levels of the vitamin are lowered by both physiological and psychological stress and that those with chronic diseases should probably have increased intakes. Because of the collagen production necessary for healing wounds, maintaining an adequate C level is particularly important in times of illness; thus, therapeutic doses are often used to treat burn patients and those who have undergone surgery. A study performed in England even suggests that bed-sores of chronically ill patients may heal faster with extra vitamin C.

A study similar to Anderson's, performed by Coulehan and his colleagues at a Navajo boarding school, similarly showed no difference in the number of respiratory illnesses. However, among the younger children in the study there were 26 percent fewer days of illness in the vitamin group; among older girls taking the vitamin there were 33 percent fewer days. No difference was shown among older boys.

While studies of this type and magnitude are replete with problems (not the least of which is the subjective nature of determining the severity of symptoms), Anderson has suggested that the differences in results may have to do with the initial nutritional status of the subjects in such trials. "Thus," he says, "it seemed possible that the differences between the first Toronto and Arizona studies might be due to the fact that one group consisted of urban, well-nourished adults, while the other consisted of young, possibly less well-nourished school children on an Indian reservation."

What it boils down to is the fact that those who already maintain tissue saturation levels of the vitamin are probably less likely to benefit by increased vitamin C intake. Anderson and others are of the opinion that maintaining tissue saturation—as do animals that produce their own C—is probably not a bad policy. He also feels, however, that in light of present knowledge, intake of C should probably be limited to the amount necessary to maintain saturation. As mentioned, for most people, 100 to 150 mg a day should be more than sufficient. That is usually an increase easily met in the diet.

Even if there weren't still disagreement about the amount of vitamin C we need to obtain optimum nutrition, which there is, the storm would continue to rage over the value of pharmacological doses of this vitamin. Name a disease—colds, arthritis, cancer, atherosclerosis, mental illness, diabetes, allergies, etc.—and someone has probably promoted megadoses of vitamin C as its cure. Some of the claims are outright nonsense, others are interesting theories that have not proven out in testing, and still others present hopeful possibilities. Reams have been written about the implications for megadoses of vitamin C, so it certainly is not possible to explore all of the claims and evidence here, but it seems worthwhile to briefly touch on a few of the more promising possibilities for the vitamin.

The role of vitamin C in the prevention and/or cure of cancer is one area of research currently receiving a great deal of attention. As an active reducing agent, ascorbic acid has been shown to inhibit nitrosamine formation in vitro. As we know, nitrosamines are powerful carcinogens possibly formed from the nitrites used to cure meats. Ascorbic acid is now commonly added to some products to block nitrosamine formation.

Because ascorbic acid acts as an anti-oxidant (a substance that reacts with an oxidizing agent and effectively disables it so it cannot attack more fragile molecules), some scientists believe it may play a key role in cancer prevention by inhibiting oxidation of suspect chemicals. The vitamin showed promise in lowering the incidence of malignant tumors in the bladders of both men and animals.

In some cases ascorbic acid has been used with success as a chemopreventative in the treatment of precancerous conditions. A pilot study showed regression of rectal polyps in four of five patients (all polyps disappeared in two patients) with familial polyposis when treated with 3 grams of C daily for four to thirteen months. Patients with polyposis have a very high risk of developing cancer of the colon. According to the National Cancer Institute, a large clinical trial is now underway to determine whether daily doses of vitamin C can prevent colon cancer in patients with this inherited condition.

Ascorbic acid has also been suggested for use in cancer treatment as a palliative (an agent to lessen pain and severity without curing) and life-prolonging drug in cases of terminal cancer. In a non-randomized study conducted by Cameron and Campbell, patients with advanced cancer were administered 10 grams of ascorbic acid per day. Their progress—and that of 50 other test subjects who had received radiation and chemotherapy prior to the ascorbate treatment—was measured against that of one thousand patients whose histories were selected from the records of a Scottish hospital. The mean survival of the patients given ascrobic acid was 210 days, as compared to fifty days for the selected controls. In a revised version of the study. Cameron and Pauling found that the mean survival of patients given vitamin C was greater than 293 days, as compared with thirty-eight days for the controls."

Because of the bias possible in non-randomized studies using selected controls, a randomized, controlled, double-blind trial was later conducted by Creagan and his associates at the Mayo Clinic under the sponsorship of the National Cancer Institute. To evaluate the effectiveness of vitamin C in relieving the symptoms and extending the lifespan of patients with advanced cancer who could no longer benefit from standard therapy, doctors there randomly divided 150 patients into two groups. One group received 10 grams per day of ascorbic acid, the other a comparably flavored placebo. The conclusion of the researchers? "We were unable to demonstrate any statistically significant benefit of high-dose vitamin C in selected patients with advanced cancer."

According to Robert J. Avery, Jr. of the National Cancer Institute, "Vitamin C did not improve survival time and in terms of statistical significance, vitamin C had no greater effect than a placebo in causing side effects, such as nausea and vomiting, or improving symptoms, such as pain and poor appetite. However, in spite of this, the number of treated patients experiencing pain relief and increasing strength was greater than the number of control (placebo) patients experiencing these symptomatic effects."

As the researchers who conducted the Mayo Clinic study point out, however, only nine of their subjects had not previously received chemotherapy or radiation therapy, whereas none of the patients in the Cameron/Campbell study had received such traditional treatment. "It is therefore impossible," says the Mayo Clinic report, "to draw any conclusions about the possible effectiveness of vitamin C in previously untreated patients. In Cameron and Campbell's report of a 10 percent regression rate in 50 patients with widely disseminated cancer, none had received definitive prior treatment and presumably were more immunocompetent than our patients. Since vitamin C may have an impact on host resistance to cancer, we recognize that earlier immunosuppressive treatment might have obscured any benefit provided by this agent. Nevertheless, the non-randomized study that showed a fourfold enhancement of survival with vitamin C included patients who had received conventional cancer treatment (i.e., cytotoxic agents and radiation therapy). This improvement could not be substantiated by our study."

Another study to determine the effectiveness of vitamin C therapy in cancer patients is currently underway at the Mayo Clinic. Patients with cancer of the colon or rectum who have had no previous chemotherapy or radiation therapy and who have advanced disease with minimal symptoms will be eligible for this study. The investigation has just begun and results will not be available for several years.

But cancer and the cold aren't the only diseases against which vitamin C's effectiveness has been tested. Following is a very brief rundown of tentative results from other areas of research; unfortunately, most of them are as inconclusive and confusing as those obtained from studies of the vitamin's effect on cancer and the common cold.

Some studies have shown vitamin C capable of lowering serum lipid levels (high levels are a recognized factor in heart disease and stroke), while other studies have actually shown lipid levels to be unaffected or increased!

While findings are premature, future studies may substantiate current evidence that vitamin C could have a therapeutic effect on heart disease through its role in preventing and/or reducing atherosclerotic lesions of the arteries, by promoting the health of blood vessels, and by protecting the heart muscle itself by affecting the ability of its cells to survive a poor blood supply. According to Anderson however, "It must be reemphasized that these intriguing theoretical speculations and isolated favourable (sic) reports should not be accepted, uncritically, to justify indiscriminate vitamin C therapy in heart disease, but should rather be used as the starting point for precise and well-designed studies."

According to Brody, "vitamin C in megadose formulations has been used—sometimes successfully—to treat a number of disorders. These include disorders of collagen synthesis and osteogenesis imperfecta, an abnormality of bone development." Another report points out vitamin C's effectiveness in dissolving gallstones.

Results in some areas have been promising, but, as has been emphasized over and over again, they are far from conclusive. As *The Vitamin Book* says, "the Food and Drug Administration Advisory Panel on Vitamin and Mineral Drug Products for Over-the-Counter Human Use concluded that controlled clinical studies do not support the claims for using vitamin C to treat atherosclerosis (hardening of the arteries), allergy, mental illnesses including schizophrenia, corneal ulcers, thrombosis (blood clots), or pressure sores." Runners will also be disappointed to know that large quantities of C have no proven effect in improving athletic performance.

TOXICITY

Some avenues of research regarding the therapeutic use of vitamin C hold promise; but, at present, unfortunately, too many of them reach dead ends. While many people might feel safer exceeding the RDA slightly to attain tissue saturation levels of the vitamin (attainable with just 100 to 150 mg per day), in light of current evidence—and potential toxicity—megadoses of the vitamin are not advisable for the average person.

On the advice of Pauling and others, many Americans are taking vitamin C in quantities exceeding one gram (1000 mg) per day. In fact, doses ranging from 5000 to 10,000 mg are not uncommon. While it is true that vitamin C in excess of that required to saturate the tissues is eventually excreted in the urine, evidence continues to mount that all that ascorbic acid may be causing some trouble before it finds its way out of the body.

Doses of vitamin C of a few hundred milligrams or so show very little toxicity. But as doses increase to 1000 milligrams or more, there begins to be cause for concern. Among the milder symptoms of vitamin C overdose are gastrointestinal problems, including diarrhea and abdominal cramps. Megadoses can acidify the urine and cause a burning sensation during urination and raise oxalic and uric acid levels, possibly increasing the chances of kidney stones and gout in susceptible individuals. A study by Dr. Victor Herbert reports that quantities of C may destroy vitamin B12, resulting in serious deficiencies. Other studies have challenged his findings, however. At the same time, though, C increases the absorption of iron, which could mean an excess for some people. Urinary levels of calcium and sodium are also affected.

Hayes and Hegsted report that as little as 400 mg of C a day in the diets of pregnant women can result in infants with rebound scurvy. While in the uterus, the metabolic system of the fetus adjusts to excessive amounts of vitamin C being ingested by the mother by speeding up excretion. After birth, when the infant is consuming only normal amounts of vitamin C, the excretion mechanism continues to work overtime, carrying out even the C the child needs to maintain normal serum and tissue levels. The unfortunate result: infantile scurvy. While excessive doses of C are not advised for anyone, pregnant and lactating women should be especially wary of megadoses, as the doses do not have to be that large to adversely affect an infant, and millions of Americans today are routinely taking doses in the 500- to 1500-milligram range. Vitamin C dependency and/or rebound scurvy can occur in adults, also, when megadoses of C are stopped abruptly. Dr. Herbert suggests tapering off megadoses by about 10 to 20 percent daily.

Finally, megadoses of vitamin C can interfere with the results of lab tests used to diagnose illness. C, for example, can change the results of blood tests and cause false negative and false positive results in urine sugar tests. C can also cause false-negative results in blood-in-stool tests used to diagnose such disorders as cancer of the colon. The vitamin may also hinder the diagnosis of liver disease. If you are taking large quantities of C, advise your physician before undergoing any lab tests.

One last note of caution is in order: attempting to treat yourself with vitamins for serious illnesses (i.e., cancer, heart disease, etc.) on the basis of tests with animals and unsubstantiated claims, can be extremely hazardous by delaying diagnosis and proper treatment that could save your life.

RDA AND AVAILABILITY

As has already been pointed out, the RDA for vitamin C is aimed at maintaining a body pool of 1500 mg of the vitamin. According to the 1980 RDA report, "A pool of this magnitude will protect against overt signs of scurvy in the adult male for a period of 30-45 days....Although there is some evidence that larger intakes, approximating 200 mg/day, may produce a larger body pool...the Committee on Dietary Allowances believes that efforts to attain such a pool size are unnecessary in view of the decreased efficiency of absorption and increased rate of excretion of unmetabolized ascorbic acid at these higher intakes." To maintain a 1500 mg body pool size, the RDA for vitamin C has been set at 60 mg (up from 45 mg in the 1974 RDAs) for most adults. Pregnant and lactating women get an additional 20 and 40 mg, respectively. Just as an interesting note, the Dietary Standards for Canada (and many other countries), set the recommended intake at 30 mg with no apparent ill effects.

Thanks to James Lind, most of us think of vitamin C in terms of citrus fruits, and oranges, lemons, grapefruit, limes, tangerines, and so on, are indeed an excellent source. A single glass of orange juice, for example, easily exceeds the body's requirement for the entire day. Tomatoes, broccoli, greens, cantaloupes, strawberries and other fruits and vegetables are also very fine sources. Although vitamin C is one of the most fragile of the vitamins, subject to loss in storage and preparation, it is still relatively simple to exceed the RDA for this vitamin by making fresh fruits and vegetables an indispensable part of the diet.

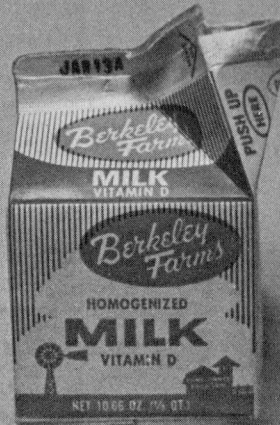

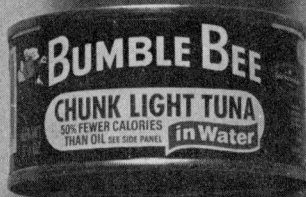

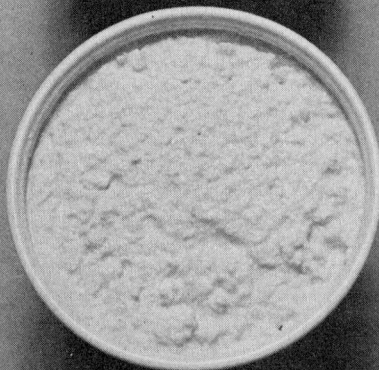

14

Vitamin D

FORM AND FUNCTION

When Sir Edward Mellanby began his work on rickets in the early 1900s, the disease had reached epidemic proportions in his native England; indeed, some estimates indicate that rickets afflicted as many as 90 percent of the children in Europe. Mellanby managed to induce the disease in dogs maintained on a diet of oatmeal. Because foods that were known to contain McCollum's Fat Soluble A cured Mellanby's test animals, he concluded that A was the antirachitic vitamin. McCollum, however, was not so sure about the role of A in rickets. With the use of heat and oxygen, he destroyed the vitamin A content of cod liver oil and found that it nonetheless contained a substance that cured rickets. He backed up these findings by curing rickets with coconut oil, which has no vitamin A content. Credited with its discovery in 1922, McCollum called the new fat-soluble vitamin D.

In the meantime, other researchers had made the interesting discovery that children with rickets could be cured simply by exposing them to sunlight or artificial ultraviolet light. Puzzled, other scientists examined the livers of both rachitic rats that had been irradiated and those that had not. When it was found that the former contained the antirachitic factor vitamin D, it was learned that animals have a substance that can be changed to vitamin D by ultraviolet light. Further, it was found that irradiation of food could also produce the antirachitic vitamin. As Dr. H.F. DeLuca notes, "These important discoveries led to the use of ultraviolet light irradiation of such foods as milk and butter to fortify them with vitamin D and thus eliminate rickets as a major medical problem." Vitamin D was isolated and chemically identified in 1931.

There are two forms of vitamin D, which seem to have equal activity in man. Vitamin D2 or ergocalciferol is the form that results when a plant sterol, ergosterol (found in molds and yeast), receives ultraviolet irradiation. Vitamin D3 or cholecalciferol is the type formed when sunlight or artificial ultraviolet light reacts with provitamin D3 or 7-dehydrocholesterol, an oil in the skin.

Once vitamin D's sunshine connection was discovered it became clear why rickets was most prevalent in temperate (as opposed to tropical) climates, in cities, among the poor and among children born in the fall or winter. Kreutler provides an interesting perspective on the disease:

> "Because their diets contained little meat or milk, the urban poor were more likely to be afflicted. Because they spent little time out of doors, and because city streets are more often shaded, city dwellers generally received less sunlight. And because of shorter days, weaker sunlight, and colder weather, infants born in the fall or winter were kept indoors and wore more clothing when out of doors during the most crucial early bone-developing period of life. We know now, too, that the rapid spread of rickets in northern European cities in the nineteenth century was one of the results of the industrial revolution, which removed people from the sunny open spaces of the countryside and put young children to work inside homes and factories. Even for those city dwellers who spent time outdoors, ultraviolet light was largely filtered out by the smoke from coal and wood fires."

Vitamin D is absorbed in the jejunum, the middle portion of the small intestine between the duodenum and the ileum. As a result of hydroxylation in first the liver and then the kidneys, vitamin D is converted to its most biologically active form, 1, 25-dihydroxycholecalciferol, less cumbersomely known as DHCC. It has been suggested that vitamin D might be more accurately termed a prohormone than a vitamin, because, as Kreutler points out, "It can be totally synthesized in the body and because it exerts its metabolic effect only after being hydroxylated to two more active forms, HCC and DHCC. These substances fulfill the definition of hormones: synthesis in one tissue of the body, from which they are transported through the blood to another tissue where they exercise their specific effect."

Rather limited vitamin D storage occurs in the liver and fatty tissues, as well as in the brain and bones.

Vitamin D puts all of its energy, it seems, into the formation and maintenance of bones and teeth. Vitamin D begins its job by aiding in the absorption of both calcium and phosphorus. The vitamin accomplishes this task by participating in the synthesis of binding proteins that transport these essential minerals across cell membranes. Vitamin D also participates in the actual process of depositing calcium and phosphorus in the bones to give them the strength they need to support the body. At the same time, however, it is also the job of D to stimulate the production of hormones to pull calcium and phosphorus from the bones when they are needed to maintain the correct serum levels of these minerals. According to Kreutler, "Vitamin D also appears to increase re-absorption of phosphorus and calcium by the kidney and prevents excretion of phosphorus in the urine. Thus, the overall effect of vitamin D is to provide the optimal amounts of calcium and phosphorus needed for bone mineralization by increasing their availability through increased absorption and preventing the loss of phosphorus in the urine."

DEFICIENCY

With all of vitamin D's activity tied up in the building of bones, it is little wonder that deficiency of the vitamin results in the bone diseases rickets (in children) and osteomalacia (in adults). Without the minerals calcium and phosphorus to lend their strength, bones, in the case of rickets, remain soft and deform easily under the body's weight. Thus, common signs of the disease in children are bowed legs, knock-knees, spinal curvature, narrow pelvis and potbelly appearance, and often flat feet and stunted growth. Other characteristics of the disease are a protruding sternum sometimes referred to as "pigeon breast," rounded protrusions on the ribs known as rachitic rosary, deformed skull, malformed teeth susceptible to decay, and eventually muscle weakness and nervous irritability.

In adults, vitamin D deficiency manifests itself as osteomalacia. This disease is characterized by loss of calcium from the bones, which makes them weak and easily broken. The disease is accompanied by deformities, pain, weakness and difficulty in walking. Rickets is no longer common in this country (though it is still prevalent in parts of the world), but osteomalacia is, particularly among shutins and the elderly, who often don't drink milk and get very little exposure to the sun. Synthesis of the vitamin can also be a problem for blacks in northern climates, as heavily pigmented skin can prevent up to 95 percent of ultraviolet radiation from reaching the deeper layers of skin where vitamin D is synthesized.

A deficiency of vitamin D is particularly critical during infancy, childhood and adolescence, when bones and teeth are being formed. To assure that most children get enough of the vitamin at this important time, most milk today is fortified with vitamin D so that one quart contains the RDA for infants and children. Milk was the chosen vehicle for vitamin D supplementation for several reasons, the two most important of which are: 1) It is consumed in large amounts by most infants and children, 2) It contains the essential bone-building minerals calcium and phosphorus, without which vitamin D would be of little use. Because few foods other than fatty fish and fish liver oils and fortified products contain significant quantities of vitamin D, it is difficult for children and pregnant and lactating women who do not consume dairy products to get enough of the vitamin.

Secondary vitamin D deficiency may result from certain liver, kidney and endocrine disorders, from any disease that interferes with fat absorption, and from certain drugs (i.e., mineral oil, barbiturates, anticonvulsants, etc.).

WHAT CAN IT DO?

Vitamin D can prevent and/or cure bone diseases (i.e., rickets, osteomalacia) caused by a deficiency of the vitamin. It cannot, however, reverse the permanent damage of such diseases. Also, much of vitamin D's job consists of helping us to utilize calcium; it cannot prevent or cure bone diseases when calcium is absent from the diet.

In the presence of liver or kidney disease that prevents hydroxylation of vitamin D to its active forms, a condition known as vitamin D-resistant rickets may occur. Such conditions, which respond unsatisfactorily to massive doses of vitamin D, appear to be remedied by administration of a synthetic analog of the vitamin's biologically active form. Vitamin D is not effective against arthritis.

TOXICITY

Vitamin D builds strong bones, but in the absence of a deficiency, more vitamin D doesn't build *stronger* bones. Oil-soluble and capable of storage in the liver and fatty tissues, vitamin D is one of the vitamins that can be toxic in excess. Perhaps vitamin D's trouble is that it is just too conscientious. When too many vitamin D molecules show up on the job, none of them opt to take off early. Instead, they all stay, doing what they're supposed to be doing: increasing the absorption of calcium, performing the task of mineralization, and keeping up the serum calcium level. Unfortunately, all that extra calcium in the blood (hypercalcemia) isn't good for us because it has to go somewhere....and that somewhere is usually the kidneys, lungs, heart, blood vessels, etc. Aside from calcification of bones and soft tissues, hypervitaminosis D can result in nausea, loss of appetite, weight loss, weakness, aches, stiffness, polyuria (excessive urination), high blood pressure, headache, acidosis, and so on. Kidney failure can result from the excessive intake and may result in death.

The Committee on Nutrition of the American Academy of Pediatrics has determined 1000 to 3000 IU per kilogram of body weight to be dangerous, but Kreutler contends that "Sensitive infants may develop hypercalcemia on an intake of 1800 to 2000 IU per day, since the toxicity threshold is only four to five times the RDA." Individuals vary greatly in their sensitivity to the vitamin.

While the danger of excessive intake of pill-form supplements may be obvious, some people, including the late, revered Adelle Davis, are under the impression that the vitamin, as it occurs naturally, is non-toxic. That is not the case and, in fact, most cases of hypervitaminosis D are attributable to excessive intake of cod liver oil, which carries a whopping 1275 IU of the vitamin in a single tablespoon!

RDA AND AVAILABILITY

Until recently the Recommended Daily Allowances of vitamin D were listed in international units (IU), which is defined as the activity contained in 0.025 mcg of cholecalciferol or vitamin D3. Now, however, the RDAs are expressed as micrograms of cholecalciferol. At 10 mcg (400 IU), RDAs for infants, children and adolescents are double those for most adults. The recommended intake for pregnant and lactating women is also set at 10 mcg.

As noted, most foods are rather poor sources of vitamin D, with the exception of fatty fish (tuna, salmon, herring, shrimp, etc. are rich in the vitamin), eggs, liver and butter. Milk, as we know, is a good source only when fortified with the vitamin, which it usually is. According to McGill and Pye, "Because of the toxic effect of too much vitamin D, the fortification of foods other than milk with this vitamin is under review by the Food and Drug Administration."

The decreased needs of most adults for vitamin D can probably be easily met by exposure to sunlight. Further, overexposure to the sun, while painful and harmful in other regards, cannot result in hypervitaminosis D. Those who do not have regular exposure to the sun (office workers, etc.), or live in adverse climates or where pollution is heavy, can still easily meet their needs with attention to the foods they consume or the addition of milk to the diet. In cases where commercial supplements are used, their potency should never exceed the RDA.

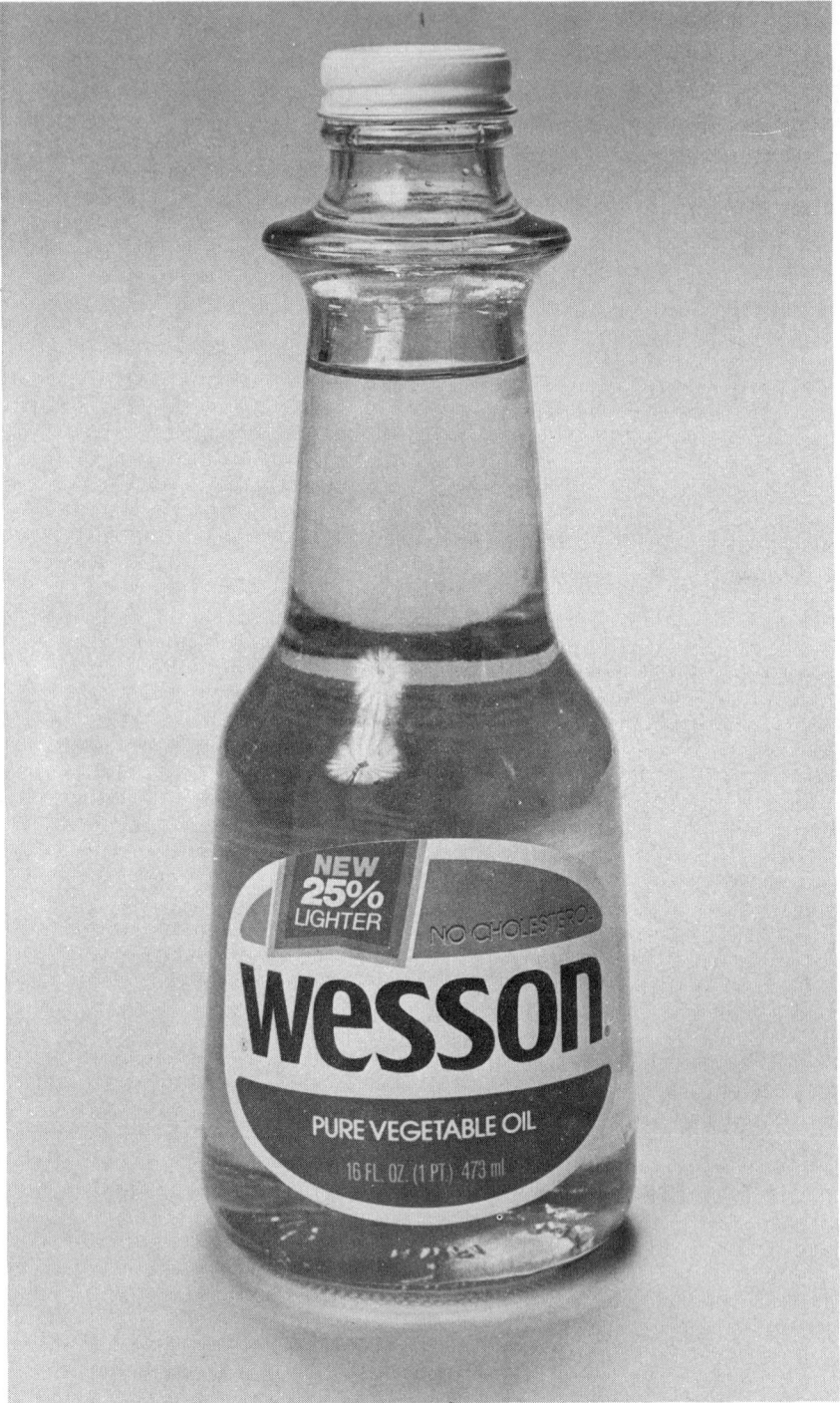

15

Vitamin E (Tocopherol)

FORM AND FUNCTION

One need only go back to the discovery of vitamin E to find the source of its reputation as the "sex vitamin," capable of maintaining or restoring virility and fertility. The vitamin's existence first came to light in 1922 when H.M. Evans and K.S. Bishop at the University of California, Berkeley, found that a purified diet severely affected the reproductive ability of rats. Male rats became sterile and females resorbed their fetuses or gave birth to deformed or stillborn offspring. The addition of certain foods to the diet—later learned to contain vitamin E—even as late as one-third through the pregnancy, prevented or reversed reproductive problems. These dramatic findings resulted in the new vitamin's name, tocopherol (from the Greek *tokos*, "childbirth," and *phero*, "to bring"), and its reputation—unearned in man—for fertility. Vitamin E was isolated from wheat germ oil in 1936 and synthesized in 1938.

Vitamin E occurs in a number of natural and synthetic forms, including alpha-tocopherol, beta-tocopherol, gamma-tocopherol, delta-tocopherol, and the tocotrienols. Alpha-tocopherol is the most common and biologically active form, with the other forms assumed to have anywhere from 1 to 50 percent of its activity. Absorbed in the small intestine in much the same way as other oil-soluble vitamins, E is transported in the blood by lipoproteins. While some storage takes place in the liver, muscles and adrenal and pituitary glands, most vitamin E is stored in the fatty tissues. According to "A Scientific Status Summary by the Institute of Food Technologists' Expert Panel on Food Safety & Nutrition and the Committee on Public Information," "As much as several grams of the tocopherols may be stored in the body and they are only slowly eliminated; this may account for the difficulty of finding positive evidence of deficiencies."

Kreutler notes the somewhat limited efficiency of vitamin E absorption when she points out that "only 50 to 85 percent of the dietary intake of this vitamin actually enters the bloodstream." For those believers in vitamin E's remarkable curative powers who are taking huge supplements of this vitamin, the following observation by Kreutler might also be interesting: "Efficiency of absorption is....impaired as intake increases. Tissue levels of vitamin E only double when intake is increased to ten times the RDA for the vitamin. For this reason, those who take megadoses of vitamin E are surely getting less than anticipated for their money."

It has been difficult to determine exactly what vitamin E does because the virtual non-existence of a deficiency in humans has made it difficult to determine what a *lack* of it does....or doesn't do. Probably one of the most clearly defined functions of vitamin E is as an anti-oxidant. In this role vitamin E reacts with oxidizing agents or free radicals capable of causing damage to other more fragile molecules and effectively disables them. In this way it may play a major role in protecting other oxygen-sensitive nutrients like vitamin A, polyunsaturated fatty acids (used to build cell membranes, etc.) and other cell membrane constituents, and some enzymes. Like vitamin C, E can help guard against nitrosamine formation. Because of its anti-oxidant capabilities, vitamin E has been used as a preservative in foods.

Vitamin E may play an important role in many more less understood functions and is thought, according to Kreutler, to "be required, although in minute amounts, for the synthesis of heme (a part of the hemoglobin molecule and of other metabolically essential body chemicals)."

DEFICIENCY

Because of its wide availability in foods and large body reserves, producing a vitamin E deficiency in humans takes some work. One study that attempted to induce clinical deficiency of vitamin E was performed at the Elgin State Hospital in Illinois between 1953 and 1961. Maintained on a diet almost entirely devoid of vitamin E (removing the vitamin E content from foods is a difficult and costly procedure), patients, after 20 months, still exhibited blood levels of vitamin E that were 50 percent of those of patients fed the same diet with vitamin E added. It took two to three years for any biochemical changes to occur and these consisted only of a slight decrease in the lifespan of red blood cells. There were, however, no manifestations of anemia and the subjects developed no symptoms.

Almost all evidence of vitamin E deficiency has been seen in premature infants because of their reduced absorption of fat. According to Kreutler, "Low serum levels are found in newborns generally but rise within the first month of life, especially in breast-fed full-term infants. There are reports of deficiency symptoms— irritability, edema, and hemolytic anemia (caused by the destruction of red blood cells by oxidation)—in premature infants fed a commercial formula with inadequate vitamin E content; these symptoms were reversed when vitamin E was administered."

Deficiency of E can also occur in adults who have an impaired ability to absorb dietary fat. The problem occurs most often among post-gastrectomy patients and those with cystic fibrosis, liver cirrhosis, obstructive jaundice, pancreatic insufficiency, and sprue (a chronic tropical disease characterized by anemia and gastrointestinal disorders). According to Dr. J.G. Bieri of the National Institute of Health, however, "In these patients, although blood levels of the vitamin may be very low, no symptomatology which responds to vitamin E has been observed. Life span of their red cells is often shortened but anemia is not found. A few cases of muscle damage have been noted histologically, but generally muscle function is not impaired." Thus, although vitamin E is involved in several important functions, when it is in short supply, no dramatic symptoms like those associated with deficiencies of the other vitamins develop. It's not surprising, then, that vitamin E has often been described as a vitamin looking for a deficiency disease.

WHAT CAN IT DO?

Perhaps because no one can exactly pinpoint what a deficiency of vitamin E does to human beings, the vitamin has been promoted as an effective agent against just about every ill known to modern man. In fact, says *The Vitamin Book*, there are "60 conditions for which the vitamin had been recommended as a preventive, treatment or cure." While many of these claims come from out of the blue, others are extrapolated from results of studies with animals. The experiment with infertile rats that gave vitamin E its reputation as the sex vitamin is probably the best example. But, for one thing, the kind of severe deficiency that resulted in the disorder in those test animals does not even appear to be reproducible in humans. For another, scientific research does not bear out any of the claims for vitamin E in increasing fertility or sexual endurance or facilitating normal pregnancy. Due to the psychological nature of sexuality, experimental results in this area are extremely susceptible to the placebo effect.

A common claim for vitamin E is that it is a useful treatment for muscular dystrophy. This claim, too, is based on studies with animals in which they developed symptoms resembling those of muscular dystrophy in humans. Extensive testing has shown the vitamin to have no effect upon this genetic disease in humans.

A study in which an E-deficient diet appeared to produce heart abnormalities in cows sent many physicians scurrying off to prescribe vitamin E to their patients who had had heart attacks. A number of controlled studies since that time have revealed vitamin E to have no beneficial effect in preventing or treating heart disease.

The claim that vitamin E will slow the aging process comes from its role as an anti-oxidant. Since many aspects of aging are the result of oxidative deterioration, (i.e., as Kreutler points out, "free radicals are believed to participate in the formation of 'aging pigments' which may contribute to the aging process in various tissues."), it has been theorized that vitamin E should be able to slow the process. While tests with animals have shown a lowered incidence of aging pigments with vitamin E treatment, there has been no demonstrable effect on any other aspect of aging, nor has mortality been shown to be slowed.

Vitamin E's anti-oxidant qualities have also prompted theories that it might play a role in the prevention and/or cure of certain types of cancer. Thus far, no definitive proof has been forthcoming. But one preliminary study has suggested that extra vitamin E in the diet may reduce the amount of mutagenic activity in the stool, a finding that could have implications for development of cancer of the bowel. The possibilities are intriguing, and followup studies are currently underway.

Another area where vitamin E may prove a useful anti-oxidant is against air pollution. Some very promising studies with test animals have shown that generous amounts of the vitamin can help protect lung cells from oxidative damage from pollutants such as ozone and nitrogen dioxide. The animal tests *seem* to have positive implications for similar applications in humans.

Probably of most interest to runners and other athletes are the encouraging statements made about vitamin E's ability to improve athletic performance. However, those looking for greater strength and endurance had probably better look elsewhere. Such theories have never held up under testing. One very good example is a well-controlled study by Sharman and his colleagues. The Institute of Food Technologists' report describes it succinctly:

> "Two groups of 13 boarding-school boys each were studied. Each boy was given either 400 mg of vitamin E or a placebo daily during a period of six weeks in which they were training in swimming. Evaluation of the effect of vitamin E was conducted with a battery of tests, including measurements of muscular development, heart and lung efficiency, and muscle fitness and coordination. As was expected, the athletic training itself significantly improved individual physiological function and performance, but there was no significant additional effect of vitamin E."

Vitamin E has acquired such an enviable reputation over the years that we even apply it to our bodies externally, in the hope that it will heal scars, stop aging, and beautify our skin. Health food, drug and grocery store shelves are well-stocked with E-containing shampoos, creams, lotions, salves and oils, but there is no evidence to prove the vitamin's value in these kinds of applications, either.

Is vitamin E good for anything then? E, like the other vitamins, is an important nutrient with very specific and very necessary functions in the body. Whether it also proves a useful drug largely remains to be seen. But there is already strong evidence that vitamin E may be a useful treatment for intermittent claudication (a circulatory problem that causes painful cramps in the calves while walking), fibrocystic breast disease (painful but benign breast lumps that may make women more susceptible to breast cancer), and retrolental fibroplasia (an eye disorder of premature infants that seems to be on the increase as improved care allows more low birth weight infants to survive).

What emerges most clearly from an appraisal of vitamin E is that it is still an enigma. It is little wonder, then, that few treatises on vitamin E slip by without quoting A.L. Tappel, one of the foremost researchers in this area:

> "While few compelling uses have been found for vitamin E,

the more research is done on the substance, the more intriguing it appears. Thus, there is the nagging suspicion that there is a very important use for the vitamin and we are just not smart enough to see it."

TOXICITY

As a fat-soluble vitamin that can collect in the liver and tissues, vitamin E has the potential for toxicity, yet very few adverse effects have been reported. Of course, it is only relatively recently that megadoses of this vitamin have come into vogue, so it may be some time before its effects are clear. Although rare, reported side effects include gastrointestinal upset, including cramps and diarrhea, dry throat, headache, flushing and dizziness. There have also been reports that very large doses can have an adverse effect on coagulation of the blood, a potentially serious problem where there is a vitamin K deficiency or where patients are already taking anticoagulants. Other symptoms have been reported in test animals, but these, like potential benefits, cannot be readily applied to man. Although, as stated, no one can speak for the long term or the sensitivities of particular individuals, it seems to be the general consensus that daily doses of this vitamin under 300 IU are relatively harmless.

RDA AND AVAILABILITY

Because, in the body, it operates so closely with the polyunsaturated fatty acids, the requirement for vitamin E is based on PUFA consumption. When the diet contains more PUFAs, more E is required also. Since, however, the two are generally found together (i.e., vegetable oils, margarines, etc. are the best sources of both), the increase is almost an automatic one. Average diets of normal, healthy individuals in the U.S. supply about 0.4 mg of alpha-tocopherol per gram of PUFA. Containing a margin of safety, the RDA for E is based on a ratio of 0.6 mg alpha-tocopherol per gram of PUFA. The recommendation for adult males is 10 mg of alpha-tocopherol equivalents (i.e., total tocopherols of all forms), for adult females, 8 mg. According to the Food and Nutrition Board report, "Analyses of balanced adult diets *as consumed* indicate average daily intakes of d-alphatocopherol ranging from 7 to 9 mg. Total tocopherols may be two to three times higher, d-alpha-tocopherol equivalents range from 8 to 11 mg."

As we know, the richest sources of vitamin E are vegetable oils (wheat germ, corn, soybean, safflower, etc.) and the products that contain them. The vitamin is actually quite stable in preparation, though prolonged storage and very high heat, such as that used in deep frying, will cause oxidation. In relation to vegetable oils, foods such as grains, legumes, and vegetables have limited quantities of vitamin E. In general, animal products contain even less.

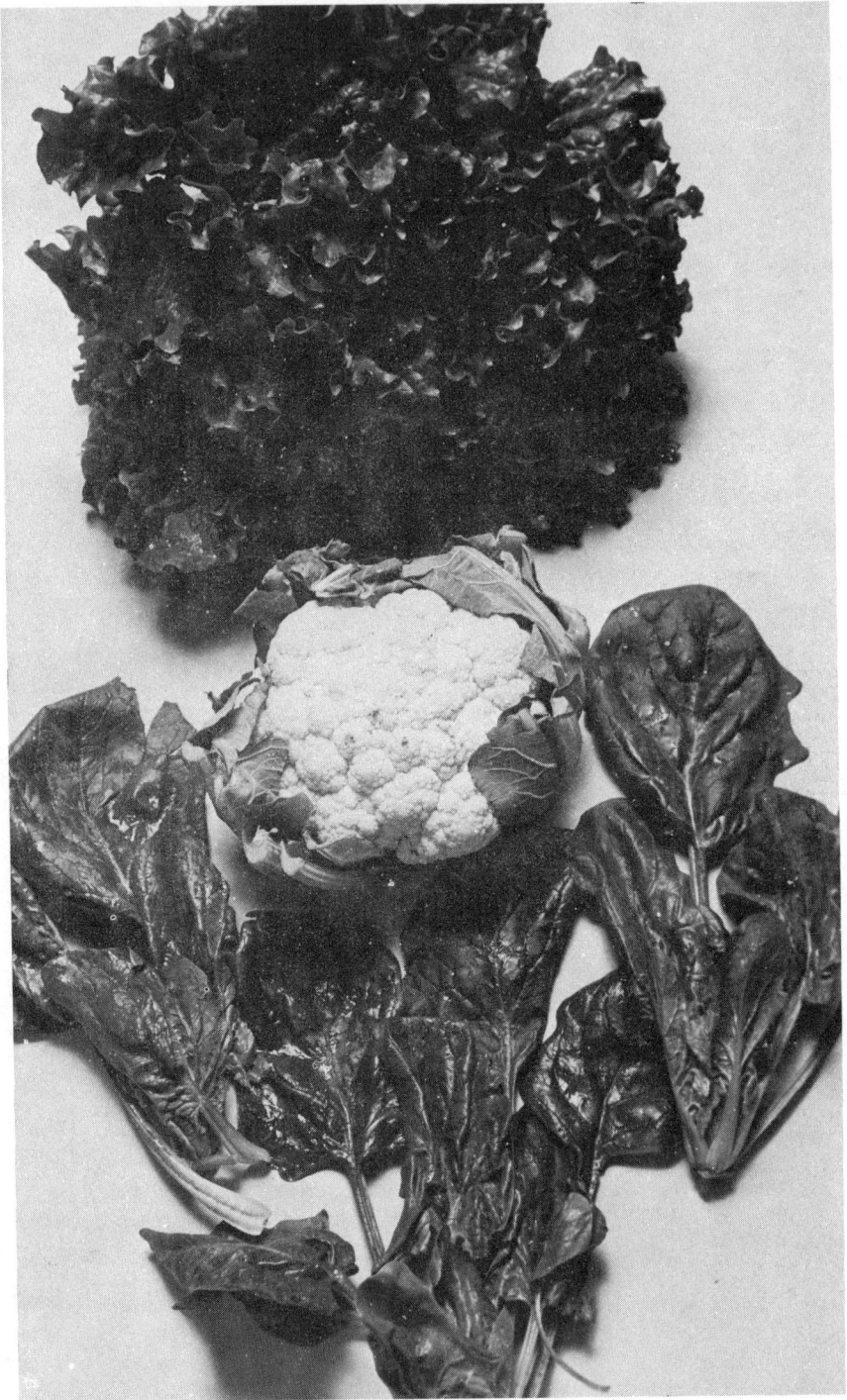

16

Vitamin K

FORM AND FUNCTION

Vitamin K was discovered by Henrik Dam, a biochemist at the University of Copenhagen, after observation of a hemorrhagic disease in newborn chicks. Dam noted that the chicks exhibited decreased levels of the blood clotting factor prothrombin and found that he could correct the condition by adding fat or alfalfa to the diet. Dam isolated the vitamin from alfalfa in 1939 and, for its anti-hemorrhagic ability, called it the "koagulationsvitamin" or vitamin K. Dam's scientific sleuthing earned him the Nobel Prize in 1943.

The term "vitamin K" comprises not one but several substances with similar biologic activity. Vitamin K1 or phylloquinone is found in green plants, while the K2 vitamins or menaquinones are present in bacteria and animals. K3 or menadione is a synthetic provitamin that is converted to menaquinone in the body. All three types are fat-soluble, but there are also water-soluble analogs or derivatives of menadione available.

Menaquinone is synthesized by bacteria in the large intestine, a source that may contribute as much as 50 to 60 percent of the body's requirement. K is absorbed in much the same way as the other fat-soluble vitamins. There is limited storage of the vitamins in the liver, skin, muscle, kidneys and heart.

Unlike some of the other vitamins, K likes to specialize. It spends all of its time involved in the synthesis of prothrombin and other substances necessary for the coagulation of blood.

DEFICIENCY

Vitamin K deficiency manifests itself as delayed blood clotting. In mild cases bleeding may continue longer than normal, while in more serious cases hemorrhaging may result. Vitamin K is plentiful in food, however, and produced in quantity in the body, so deficiency is extremely rare in the absence of elimination of the vitamin from the diet *and* malabsorption diseases or the administration of drugs that interfere with bacterial synthesis (i.e., antibiotics, sulfa drugs), act as antagonists (anticoagulants), or speed up the vitamin's elimination (i.e., some anticonvulsants).

Newborn babies do not have intestinal bacteria for the first several days after birth and vitamin K does not pass readily through the placenta, so deficiency among newborns is not uncommon. To prevent hemorrhagic disease, many hospitals rountinely administer an injection to newborns.

WHAT CAN IT DO?

Vitamin K supplements can prevent hemorrhagic disease in infants, who are often susceptible, and in persons with diseases that interfere with the vitamin's absorption. (Supplements will not work, however, where there is primary liver damage, because that is where prothrombin and other coagulants are produced). It is also sometimes administered to persons on long-term treatment with drugs that interfere with the absorption or synthesis of the vitamin. Often vitamin K is prescribed as an "antidote" when anticoagulant drugs (used in the treatment of heart disease, etc.) are too efficient.

Perhaps one of the most obvious applications that comes to mind is the treatment of hemophilia (a disease characterized by slow clotting and prolonged, uncontrolled bleeding). Unfortunately, however, as Kreutler points out, "Despite its great importance in blood clotting, administration of vitamin K has no therapeutic effect on hemophilia because this disease is caused by a genetic defect in another stage of the clotting mechanism."

TOXICITY

The phylloquinone form of vitamin K has been recommended when therapeutic use is required. But vitamin K supplementation should be undertaken *only* under the recommendation and supervision of a physician. Because of its hemolytic effect (destroying red corpuscles and releasing hemoglobin into the surrounding fluid), vitamin K3 has been prohibited from sale in over-the-counter supplements. In infants, hemolytic anemia can overload the liver, and subsequently the brain, with toxic substances. Cases of infant death have been reported.

Again, a warning is in order. Vitamin K is widely available in foods; a deficiency is highly unlikely in the absence of an interfering drug or disease. Synthetic supplements carry with them serious toxic side effects. *No one* should be taking vitamin K without the close supervision of a doctor.

RDA AND AVAILABILITY

Currently, scientists do not yet have the total picture as regards our requirements for vitamin K. An estimated requirement of 2 mcg of vitamin per kilogram of body weight has been established, but it is unclear how much of this is contributed by bacterial synthesis. As with biotin and pantothenic acid, there is no RDA, but an "estimated safe and adequate daily dietary intake." For adults this safe range is set at 70 to 140 mcg daily. The lower figure is based on the assumption that half of the daily need is supplied by bacterial synthesis; the higher the figure is based on the assumption that the entire requirement must come from the diet.

The suggested intake of vitamin K is one easily met in the U.S., where it has been estimated that the average diet contains anywhere from 300 to 500 mcg. Green, leafy vegetables (spinach, etc.) and those of the cabbage/cauliflower variety are the best sources. Meat (particularly liver) and dairy products are also adequate sources. Green—but not black—tea can, surprisingly, make a significant contribution to dietary intake of vitamin K.

PART THREE
MINERALS AND NON-VITAMINS

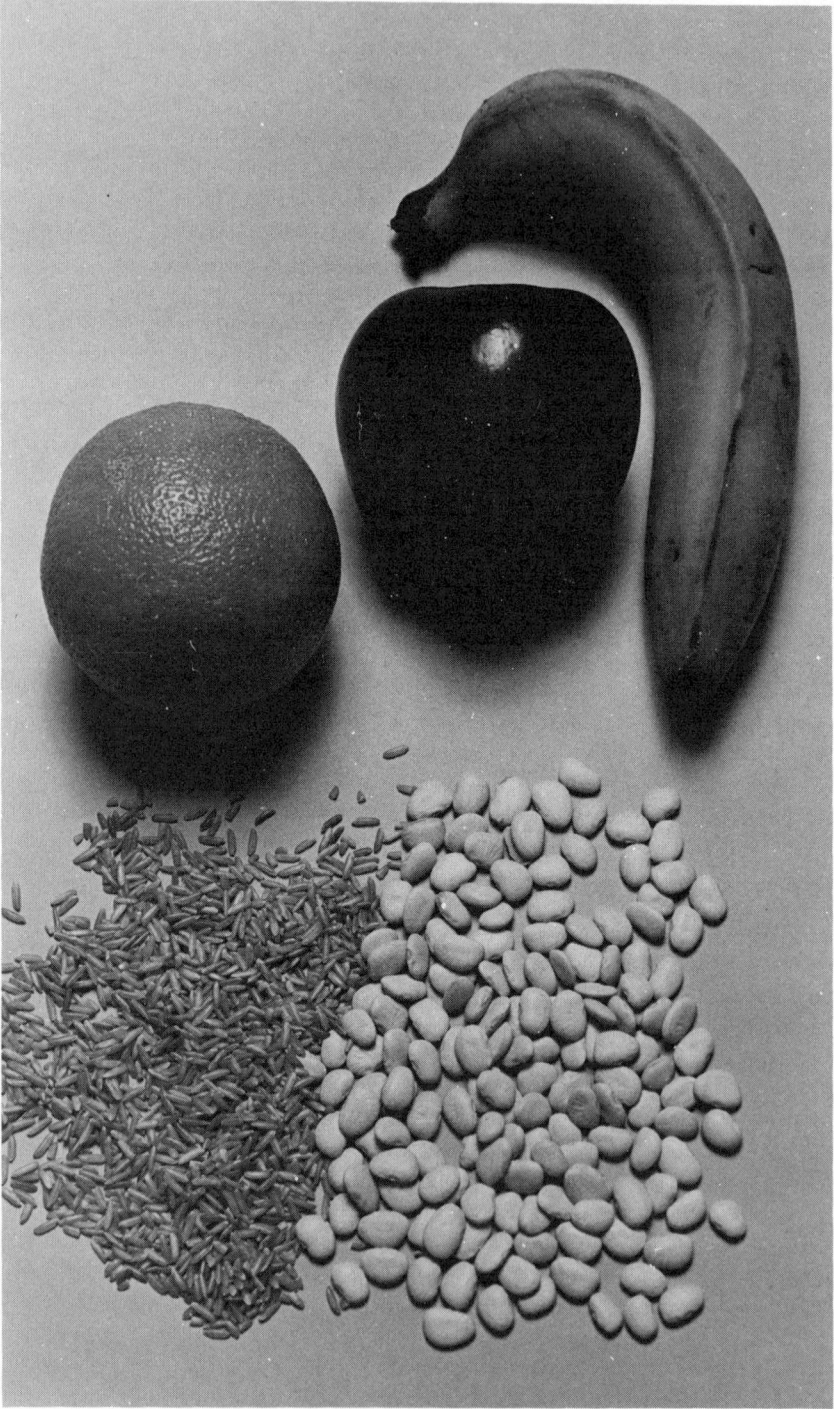

17

Non-Vitamins

A chapter on non-vitamins? That covers a lot of ground doesn't it? Afterall, anything that isn't a vitamin is a non-vitamin, right? True, but not all of those things cause as much discussion and disagreement as a select little group of non-vitamins. These are substances that either were considered vitamins at one time and are no longer, or that are not now considered vitamins but very well could be once we learn more about them. Finally, and most controversially, there are a couple of other substances that definitely are not vitamins, but that some people insist upon promoting that way. Vitamins or not, they keep cash registers across America ringing—often illegally—so they're worthy of our perusal.

To declare a substance a non-vitamin, we must have a definition of the term "vitamin." As we know, loosely defined as it is, that word is taken to mean an organic compound that is required in the diet (at least partially) in minute quantities to aid in metabolic functions and protect against specific deficiency diseases. The non-vitamin substances do not meet these requirements entirely.

Nonetheless, while there are only thirteen recognized vitamin substances, there are those who call other substances vitamins. Surprisingly, there is no law against calling other worthless or questionable substances vitamins, nor does the U.S. Food and Drug Administration have an official, *legally recognized* definition of same. The FDA does monitor such claims, however, and has won court cases that have prohibited promoters from using the "vitamin" label. As health writer Phyllis E. Lehmann points out, "The consumer's only protection is a law that prohibits making false claims directly on the package label."

Thus, despite scientific evidence, certain health food faddists and others continue to confer vitamin status on such substances as pangamic acid ("B15"), laetrile ("B17"), PABA (para-amino-benzoic acid), choline, inositol, and bioflavonoids. In his book, *The Vitamin Bible*, Earl Mindell even throws in F, G, H, L, M, P, T and U. According to the FDA, "Many companies have marketed these substances individually or in combination with essential vitamins, but consumers should not be misled by claims for them that ignore the fact that their absence from the diet does not cause a disease or any form of illness."

In the case of some of these substances—notably choline, inositol, lipoic acid, PABA, the bioflavonoids and ubiquinone—the term vitamin appears very applicable and, as already noted, it is possible that future findings might actually endow them with the coveted title. But for now, they fall short for one reason or another. Benowicz provides one explanation for their current consignment to nutritional limbo:

> "Although traditional authorities do not classify them as vitamins, at least twenty compounds exhibit vitamin or vita-minlike properties in human metabolism. Recognition may be withheld for a number of reasons having little to do with a substance's acitivity as a coenzyme. Some may be synthesized by intestinal bacteria. Others may occur so abundantly in so many foods that dietary deficiency is rare and escapes clinical detection. Yet others may yield identifiable symptoms that are difficult to relate to lack of the substance because too little of its biochemistry is fully understood. Whether such compounds are required in human nutrition is uncertain. That they are necessary for human metabolism is indisputable."

INOSITOL

As vitaminlike substances, inositol and choline are often classified with the B-complex. Inositol, whose structure closely resembles that of glucose, was first called "muscle sugar" (*inos* is the Greek for "sinews" and *ose*, of course, the suffix for sugars). Not much is clear about this substance, aside from the fact that it is a component of phospholipids (e.g., lecithin), which function in fatty acid transport, cholesterol synthesis and in the makeup of cell membranes. Inositol loses out as a vitamin primarily on the grounds that it is not required from an external source, since the human requirement is synthesized within the body. If you want more, however, there's no need to buy it in tablet form, as inositol occurs in a wide variety of foods, including fruits (particularly citrus), vegetables, legumes, nuts, grains, meat and milk.

CHOLINE

Choline has three strikes against it in the vitamin department: there is a lack of clinical and experimental evidence of choline deficiency, the body makes its own, and it is used in larger quantities than are vitamins. Like inositol, choline is a component of phospholipids. Because of its lipotropic action, which enables it to help mobilize fat stores from the liver, a deficiency of choline may be implicated in fatty liver diseases (i.e., hepatitis, cirrhosis). Choline also functions as a component of the neurotransmitter acetylcholine. "For this reason," according to Kreutler, "pharmacological doses of choline have been used to treat brain disorders that are apparently related to deficiency of choline functioning, such as tardive dyskinesia and Huntington's disease." According to the RDA report, "The average intake from foods ordinarily consumed (400-900 mg/day) is apparently adequate for health but should not be equated with a dietary requirement." If you're looking for choline in your diet, look for it with protein. Good sources are eggs, meat, grains and legumes.

BIOFLAVONOIDS

Discovered in 1936, the group of substances (rutin, hesperidin, etc.) known as the bioflavonoids was first designated vitamin P ("permeabilitats-vitamin") because it appeared to function hand in hand with ascorbic acid in decreasing capillary permeability and curing scurvy. Further studies by the father of bioflavonoids, Albert Szent-Gyorgyi, failed to confirm his earlier findings and the substance was kicked off the vitamin list. At present, the bioflavonoids, a group of yellow (*flavus*, remember, is the Latin for "yellow") pigments found in plants, have no known essential nutritional or therapeutic role, though, as Kreutler notes, they apparently have an "antioxidant effect that protects ascorbic acid from oxidative destruction." But, she adds, "this is an indirect and nonessential effect. At present there is not enough evidence to include these substances among the vitamins." If the natural vitamin companies have you convinced that you need bioflavonoids with your ascorbic acid, you can kill two birds with one stone by eating an orange, whose pulp and connective tissue are rife with the stuff. Other fruits, vegetables and grains are good sources, too.

PARA-AMINOBENZOIC ACID (PABA)

As we know, PABA is a component of folic acid, but, apparently dissatisfied being *part* of a vitamin, it wants to go out on its own. Unfortunately, it doesn't seem to have the talent for it, as nobody is sure whether it can do anything all by itself, outside of promoting growth among microorganisms. PABA apparently has some fans, however, as witnessed by its proliferating presence in supplements, skin creams and shampoos. While the reason for its appearance in these products is unclear, PABA *is* an effective sunscreen (when applied to the skin) that intercepts ultraviolet rays. Food sources include liver, as well as those health food favorites: wheat germ, brewer's yeast and sunflower seeds.

LIPOIC ACID

Another substance often classified with the B-complex is lipoic acid, a sulfur-containing fatty acid that functions with other of the B vitamins in converting glucose to acetate, a critical step in energy metabolism. No one knows precisely what the bodily need for lipoic acid is, but it appears to be a small one that is easily met. Exogenous sources include liver, yeast and wheat germ.

Besides those just mentioned, there are many more substances that occur in foods; some of them have known functions in the human body and some of them do not. None of them currently meet the criteria for obtaining vitamin status. The Food and Nutrition Board, which sets the RDAs, is aware of these substances and even classifies them into the following groups: "Nutrients Known To Be Essential For Certain Higher Animals But For Which No Proof Exists For A Dietary Need By Humans" (i.e., choline, trace elements, and growth factors); "Substances In Food That Appear Sometimes To Have Essential Nutrient Activity For Higher Animals Or That May Be Acting Pharmacologically" (i.e., linoleic and arachidonic acids, taurine, caffeine, alcohol, bioflavonoids, etc.); "Substances Known To Be Growth Factors For Lower Forms Of Life But For Which No Dietary Requirement For Higher Animals Or Humans Is Known" (i.e., Coenzyme Q or ubiquinone, lecithin, lipoic acid, PABA, nucleotides and nucleic acids, etc.); and "Substances For Which No Essential Nutrient Effect Is Known In Animals, Humans, Or Lower Species." Apart from "vitamin U," orotic acid ("B13") and any other substances dubbed vitamins, chlorophyll, herbs, etc., this group encompasses two of the most controversial non-vitamins: "B15" or pangamic acid and "B17" or laetrile.

PANGAMIC ACID

Athletes in particular may be familiar with pangamic acid or pangamate, which is touted for its ability to increase tissue levels of oxygen. A particularly hot seller at the moment, pangamic acid is brought to you by the same folks who brought you laetrile and is derived from the same sources: apricot pits and other seeds (hence the name from *pan*, "all" and *gamete*, "seed"). While he asserts that, "Because its essential requirement for diet has not been proved, it is not a vitamin in the strict sense," Earl Mindell goes on to list what, based on his study of Soviet tests, B15 can do for you. The list is a long one: extend cell life span, neutralize the craving for liquor, speed recovery from fatigue, lower blood cholesterol levels, protect against pollutants, aid in protein synthesis, relieve symptoms of angina and asthma, protect the liver against cirrhosis, ward off hangovers, and stimulate immunity responses. The Russians, by the way, according to Mindell, "are thrilled with its results, while the U.S. Food and Drug Administration wants it off the market."

Reactions are strongly mixed on this substance. Its backers push it as a miracle drug that provides extra energy, dramatically improves athletic ability and cures everything from autism and alcoholism to schizophrenia and senility. Benowicz characterizes it as a coenzyme of the B-complex that is "involved in respiration, protein synthesis, and the regulation of steroid hormones. Because its principal effect is to increase blood and tissue supplies of oxygen," he says, "the vitamin may help detoxify pollutants, protect the liver, and extend life expectancy for individual cells, while promoting the activity of white blood cells and reducing susceptibility to infection."

Benowicz further contends that the FDA has ignored evidence of pangamic acid's coenzyme functions and "threatens to brand the vitamin as an 'additive' when included in food supplements." He goes on to say that "In France, Spain, Germany, Japan and the USSR, the vitamin is regarded as essential and recommended allowances have been set at levels of 25 to 50 mg/day for adults. Symptoms of toxicity appear only at dosages of 50,000 to 100,000 times greater than this amount." To the list of conditions pangamic acid can prevent or cure he adds heart disease, premature aging, allergies, mild poisoning, neuritis, hypertension, hepatitis and diabetes.

According to the Food and Nutrition Board, pangamic acid is

"an ill-defined mixture of dimethyl-glycine and sorbitol and is wrongly called vitamin B15." Dr. Victor Herbert, a member of the Board and chief of the hematology and nutrition laboratory at Bronx Veterans Administration Medical Center and professor of medicine at Downstate Medical Center in New York, says of B15: "The amusing thing is that it doesn't exist. There is no such substance. The seller takes any chemicals he chooses off the shelf, compresses them into tablets, and throws them into bottles labeled B15 or pangamic acid." According to writer Phyllis E. Lehmann, Dr. Herbert has also indicated that the "Main ingredients of the two leading brands have proven to be mutagenic—and probably carcinogenic as well. One also has caused kidney damage and birth defects in laboratory rats."

Summarizing current research on pangamic acid, Kreutler says, "Pangamate's developers have never furnished any proof (other than testimonials) of its vitamin properties and curative powers. Nevertheless, it is widely used in the Soviet Union and in a number of European and other countries. Claims made for it by the Soviets include maintenance of tissue levels of oxygen, and this would seem to accord with claims made for its energy-giving property; however, it apparently does not increase body intake of oxygen but, rather, removes greater amounts of oxygen from blood into tissues, which may, in fact, be hazardous rather than beneficial. ....as with Laetrile, it does not meet the criteria for a vitamin. Lacking evidence for its effectiveness as a drug or for its safety, and with the chemical makeup of various preparations in dispute, the Food and Drug Administration has refused to approve its sale as a drug or dietary supplement."

Because they derive from the same source, pangamic acid is capable of the same kind of toxicity as laetrile; but more about that when we review what is perhaps the most controversial drug of the decade.

LAETRILE

For almost thirty years, since its discovery in 1952 by biochemist Ernst T. Krebs, Jr., laetrile has been promoted as a cancer preventative and cure. But, despite such bold promises as a cure rate of 15 percent for those with advanced cancer and 80 percent for those detected early, and the prevention of cancer in 100 percent of those who are healthy now, extensive, controlled testing has shown this substance to have no effect against the disease. Despite claims by laetrile supporters (including such organizations as the Committee for Freedom of Choice in Cancer Therapy) that there is a conspiracy by the FDA and the medical establishment to cover up this cure by refusing to test it, the fact is that laetrile has received much more extensive testing than any other alleged anti-cancer agent, including some that exhibited a good deal more initial promise.

Laetrile, also known by its generic chemical name, amygdalin, occurs naturally in the pits of apricots, peaches, plums, etc. and is one of a group of closely related chemicals collectively called nitrilosides by laetrile advocates. Manufactured versions of the substance bear various trade names, including Cyto H-3 and Kemdalin. In recent years proponents have taken to calling laetrile vitamin B17.

The underlying theory upon which laetrile's alleged effectiveness against cancer is based on an involved one in which such things as "trophoblast" cells figure heavily, but, in a nutshell, the substance is purported to work this way: In addition to glucose, amygdalin contains a substance called mandelonitrile, which, in the presence of the enzyme beta-glucosidase, breaks down into the poisons benzaldehyde and cyanide. According to laetrile proponents, cancerous cells contain much more beta-glucosidase than normal cells; thus, when the drug comes in contact with these cells, the cyanide is released and the cancer cells are destroyed. Normal cells, on the other hand, are said to have not only less beta-glucosidase, but also an enzyme called rhodanese, which converts the cyanide to a harmless substance, thereby protecting normal cells.

An attractive theory....if only it were true. The fact is that only trace amounts of beta-glucosidase are found in animal tissues and there is no difference in the amount found in cancerous cells and healthy ones. Likewise, healthy tissues contain no more of the enzyme rhodanese than do cancerous tissues. According to a report on laetrile published by the American Cancer Society, "to the extent that there is any detectible difference in the levels of the enzyme beta-glucosidase in various tissues of the body, experimental evidence suggests that there is less in cancerous tissues than such organs as the liver, kidney and spleen. If Laetrile behaved in the body in accordance with the proponents' theory, the first casualties would probably be various vital organs."

Fortunately, for the vital organs of those who have undergone laetrile treatment, however, the drug does not operate according to the theory. According to Dr. David M. Greenberg, chairman and professor of biochemistry emeritus at the University of California, School of Medicine, Berkeley and San Francisco, "The tissues of the body contain such minute amounts of the enzyme beta-glucosidase, the only enzyme that can decompose laetriles, that these compounds probably are not extensively broken down when introduced parenterally (i.e. by injection) and are probably excreted mainly intact in the urine."

While nothing apparently happens when laetrile is taken by injection, oral ingestion is another story. Taken by mouth in either pill form (manufactured versions of this drug are notoriously impure, by the way) or as apricot, peach, etc. kernels, laetrile can be decomposed by beta-glucosidase present in the microbe population of the intestinal tract or in other foods, resulting in cyanide poisoning. According to the ACS report, due to the laetrile-amygdalin-vitamin B17 craze, such cases of poisoning are now being reported. In spite of laetrile's potential toxicity and the varying degrees of sensitivity among individuals, Mindell can state unequivocally that "Cumulative amounts of more than 3.0 g. can be ingested safely, but not more than 1.0 g. at any one time." He then goes on to give the *Nutrition Almanac* safe recommendation of five to thirty apricot kernels—"eaten throughout the day, but never all at the same time"—as a sufficient preventive amount. On the other hand, doctors who have treated cyanide poisoning that resulted from self-administered apricot kernels maintain: "The minimum number of seeds needed to cause disease or death is not known."

It cannot be stated strongly enough: laetrile, amygdalin, B17 or whatever you choose to call it, is toxic when taken orally; it *is not* an effective drug against cancer, nor is it, as the currently popular theory goes, a vitamin whose deficiency results in cancer. Laetrile possesses none of the qualifications necessary to call it a vitamin; it is not an essential nutrient; it does not promote any physiological process vital to the existence of any organism; no specific disease state has been linked to its lack in animals or man; and no evidence exists that cancer results from a lack of laetrile or is arrested or cured by administration of the drug.

Cancer is a terrifying disease whose conventional treatments are traumatic. For that reason its victims are easily attracted by quick, painless cures that involve no surgery, chemotherapy or radiation therapy. Unfortunately, no such easy cure currently exists. Meanwhile, tremendous progress has been made against the disease... particularly when detected in its early stages. It is unfortunately true, however, that far too many people are lured away from conventional treatment that could save their lives by the promises of drugs like laetrile. Robbing people of time, more than its potential toxicity, is the real danger of this non-vitamin.

Those who wish to know more about laetrile—the theories on which it is based, the studies performed to test its effectiveness, etc.—are advised to refer to one of the following publications:

Laetrile: Background Information (August, 1977); available from the American Cancer Society, Inc., 777 Third Avenue, New York, NY 10017 — *Laetrile: Hope—or Hoax?* by Caroline A. Zimmermann (Zebra Books, Kensington Publishing Corp., 1977).

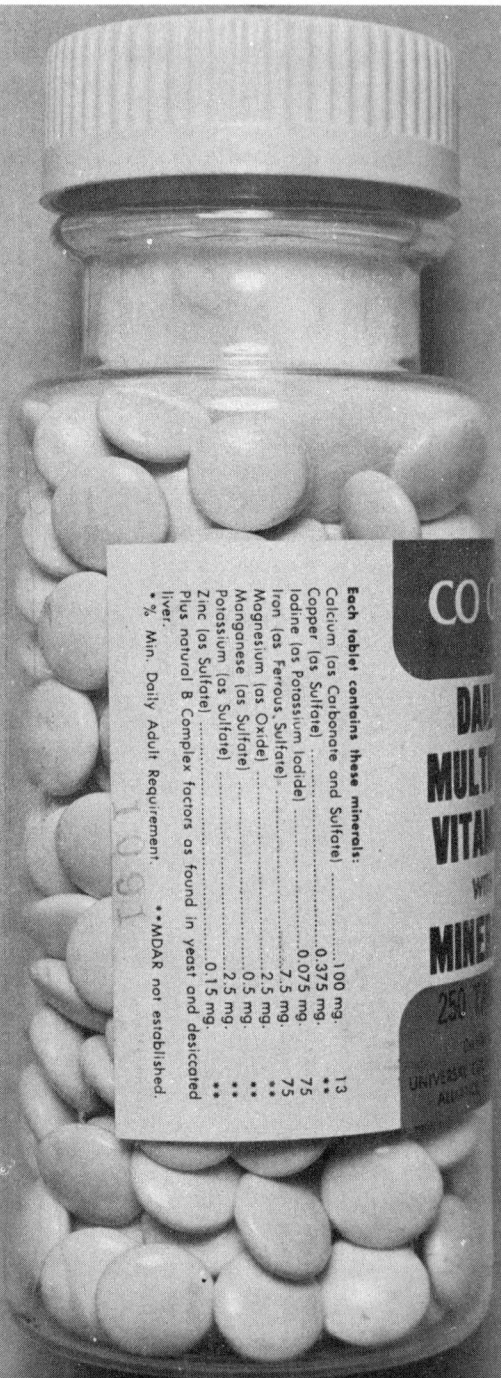

18

Minerals

The subject of dietary minerals is worthy of at least one book and probably several. We have room here for one short chapter, making it difficult to do justice to this important group of micronutrients currently at the forefront of research. Thus, the ensuing crash course is not intended to be the complete and final word on dietary minerals.

Although they are involved in an endless array of tasks in the body, the two major functions of minerals are building and regulating. Minerals are important structural elements of bones, teeth, tissues, hemoglobin, etc. They also participate in the regulation of nerve impulses, muscle contractions, enzyme reactions, fluid balance and many other functions. Without them we would not exist.

Minerals needed in relatively *large* amounts (100 milligrams or more) are called macrominerals and include calcium, phosphorus, sodium, chlorine, potassium, magnesium and sulfur. Trace minerals are required in much smaller quantities and include iron, manganese, copper, iodine, zinc, chromium, fluorine, molybdenum and selenium.

Other minerals occur in the body, as well, but there is as yet no known need for them. Some, like mercury, lead and cadmium, are toxic. Even the necessary minerals are harmful in excess. Dr. Jean Mayer has suggested that the toxic level of most minerals ranges from ten to fifty times the daily requirement, but there is evidence to suggest that even lower levels of these elements we know so little about may be toxic. An FDA report on minerals maintains that illness can result from taking the body's daily potassium requirement in a single, concentrated dose. Iron poisoning is also common among children who accidentally ingest quantities of vitamin/mineral tablets. The report goes on to say:

"Other minerals can cause adverse health effect if an individual takes as little as twice as much as is required to maintain good health. Taking too much of one essential mineral may upset the balance and function of other minerals in the body. Excess mineral intake can reduce an individual's ability to perform physical tasks and can contribute to such health problems as anemia, bone demineralization and breakage, neurological disease, and fetal abnormalities. The risks are greatest for the very young, pregnant or lactating women, the elderly, and those with inadequate diet or chronic disease. There are a number of things we do not know about the function of minerals in the body, particularly the trace elements. It is clear, however, that people who take mineral supplements should not use them in amounts greatly in excess of what the body requires."

CALCIUM

Functions: Structural element of bones and teeth (about 99 percent of the body's approximately two to three pounds of calcium is employed in this way); transmission of nerve impulses; muscle contraction (including rhythmic contraction of the heart muscle); blood coagulation; integrity of membranes and intracellular cement substances; activation of enzymes.

Deficiency: Implicated in osteoporosis, periodontal disease.

Overdose: Calcification of tissues; disturbance of delicate calcium/phosphorus ratio; impaired absorption of other minerals.

Good Sources: Milk and other dairy products, green leafy vegetables, citrus fruits, sardines, canned salmon and other fish eaten with bones, dried peas and beans.

Important Points: *The major inorganic constituent of bones and teeth is calcium phosphate, with calcium and phosphorus occurring in about equal amounts. There are differences of opinion as to the ideal calcium-to-phosphorus consumption ratio, but it is believed that optimal calcium absorption occurs when the two minerals are ingested in approximately equal amounts. A large excess of either results in imbalanced absorption and has the same effect as a calcium deficiency. The important balance of these two nutrients has been taken into account in establishing the RDAs, so they are a good guide for avoiding demineralization of bones. *Vitamin D is required for efficient absorption of calcium. *Americans receive about 60 percent of their calcium intake from milk and dairy products.*Substantial calcium loss can occur with a prolonged high-protein diet. *One quarter of all women over 65 suffer from orthopedic problems believed linked to a lifetime of inadequate calcium (the loss of calcium increases significantly with the onset of menopause).

RDA: Males 23-50: 800 mg; Females 23-50: 800 mg.

PHOSPHORUS

Functions: Structural element of bones and teeth (about 80 percent of the body's one to two pounds of phosphorus is utilized in this way), the remaining 20 percent is distributed throughout every cell in the body; necessary component of active, energy-releasing forms of some B vitamins; involved in protein synthesis within the cell; aids in absorption and transport of nutrients; helps maintain acid-base balance of blood: component of DNA and RNA.

Deficiency: Extremely rare, but may be induced by prolonged overuse of nonabsorbable antacids. Symptoms: weakness, anorexia, malaise, bone pain, demineralization of bones.

Overdose: Calcium shortage.

Good Sources: Widely distributed in foods: meat, poultry, fish, eggs, whole-grains.

Important Points: *High intake of soft drinks (which contain phosphoric acid) and processed foods with phosphate additives may contribute to an excess of this mineral in the diets of some Americans and disturb the calcium/phosphorus ratio. *The ratio of calcium to phosphorus in human milk is 2:1, in cow's milk it is 1.2:1; thus, the use of cow's milk may result in hypocalcemic tetany (severe muscle contractions and pain) in the first week of life. For that reason the infant's RDA for phosphorus is set lower than that for calcium. For all other age groups the RDAs for these minerals have been set at the same level.

RDA: Males 23-50: 800 mg; Females 23-50: 800 mg.

MAGNESIUM

Functions: Structural element of bones; activates energy-releasing enzymes; maintains electrical potential in nerves and muscle membranes.

Deficiency: May occur among alcoholics, postsurgical patients, and those with malabsorption syndromes, gastrointestinal tract diseases, and disease of the liver, kidneys or pancreas. Symptoms: tremors, convulsions, behavioral disturbances, irritability, confusion.

Overdose: Cathartic effect, potentially hazardous to those with kidney disease.

Good Sources: Whole grains, green leafy vegetables, milk and dairy products, legumes, nuts.

Important Points: *Magnesium content of processed foods is lowered considerably.

RDA: Males 23-50: 350 mg; Females 23-50: 300 mg.

SODIUM

Functions: Maintains fluid balance outside cells; transmission of nerve impulses; helps maintain acid-base balance; involved in carbohydrate and protein metabolism.

Deficiency: Extremely rare. Nausea, giddiness, muscle cramps, vomiting, circulatory failure.

Overdose: Hypertension in susceptible individuals.

Good Sources: Table salt, meat, fish, poultry, eggs, milk, processed foods.

Important Points: *Those on low-sodium diets for hypertension, etc., should check ingredient labels carefully for all forms of sodium. *The average American diet, thanks to salty snacks, processed foods, liberal sprinkling of table salt, etc., contains higher than recommended levels of sodium, a situation that can contribute to high blood pressure in susceptible individuals; blacks are particularly prone to this disorder.

Estimated Safe and Adequate Daily Dietary Intake: Adults: 1100-3300 mg.

CHLORINE

Functions: Component of hydrochloric acid, important in digestion of food in the stomach; helps maintain fluid balance outside cells; helps maintain acid-base balance of blood; enhances transport of carbon dioxide to lungs; aids in conservation of potassium.

Deficiency: Extremely rare. Since sources and regulatory system are the same as for sodium, chlorine loss usually parallels, but may greatly exceed that of sodium. Result: hypochloremic alkalosis, a disturbance of the acid-base balance.

Overdose: No known toxicity.

Good sources: Table salt (sodium chloride).

Important Points: *Those on salt-free diets for the treatment of heart, kidney, liver diseases, etc. *may* need another source of chlorine.

Estimated Safe and Adequate Daily Dietary Intake: Adults: 1700-5100 mg.

POTASSIUM

Functions: Maintains fluid balance inside cells; helps maintain acid-base balance; transmission of nerve impulses; muscle contraction; carbohydrate metabolism and protein synthesis.

Deficiency: Uncommon: may result from prolonged diarrhea or use of diuretics; has been associated with extremely inadequate protein diets in children. Symptoms: nausea, vomiting, muscle weakness, rapid heart beat, cardiac failure.

Overdose: Hyperkalemia (excess potassium in blood), occurs with kidney failure or extreme dehydration. Symptoms: muscle weakness, irregular heart beat, cardiac failure.

Good Sources: Abundant in most foods: legumes, whole grains, leafy vegetables, some fruits, meat.

Important Points: *Imbalance of electrolytes (sodium, chlorine, potassium), which can result in heart failure, is one of the dangers of fad diets that utilize diuretics or induce diarrhea. It is also a serious threat to victims of anorexia nervosa and other binge-purge eating disorders.

SULFUR

Functions: Component of amino acids, thiamin and biotin, insulin and other hormones, and keratin, the tough, fibrous protein of hair and nails.

Good Sources: High-protein foods: Meat, eggs, cheese, milk, legumes, nuts.

RDA: None established.

TRACE MINERALS

IRON

Functions: Constituent of hemoglobin necessary for tranport of oxygen to cells, where it releases energy from glucose, and for transport of resulting carbon dioxide to the lungs for excretion.

Deficiency: Iron deficiency anemia (smaller than normal red blood cells incapable of normal oxygen transport). Symptoms: weakness, tiredness, headache, pallor.

Overdose: Excess iron accumulates in soft tissues, causing cell destruction.

Good Sources: Very few foods contain iron in useful amounts. Liver is an excellent source. Other sources are meat, eggs, fish, green leafy vegetables, legumes, dried fruits, whole grains and enriched products.

Important Points: "There are approximately two thousand cases of accidental iron poisoning in the U.S. each year, mainly among children who ingest large quantities of vitamin/mineral supplements. Supplements should be kept safely out of children's reach. *More than any other vitamin or mineral, iron is the nutrient most likely to be deficient in the American diet. Groups particularly susceptible are infants, children and adolescents, who are undergoing rapid growth, women of child-bearing age due to menstrual loss of iron, and pregnant women. For the latter two groups, in particular, it is extremely difficult to meet the body's iron requirement with diet alone; supplementation is often necessary. Others likely to experience deficiencies are dieters and frequent blood donors. *Cooking in iron vessels is an easy way to get extra iron.

RDA: Males 23-50: 10 mg; Females 23-50: 18 mg.

IODINE

Functions: Component of thyroid hormones necessary for growth.

Deficiency: Goiter (thyroid gland becomes enlarged in an effort to produce adequate hormones for the body's requirement). In children: retarded physical and mental growth.

Good Sources: Iodized salt, sea foods, foods grown in coastal regions.

Important Points: *Not all salt is iodized, particularly that used in snack and convenience foods.

RDA: Males 23-50: 150 mcg; Females 23-50: 150 mcg.

OTHER NECESSARY
TRACE MINERALS

	FUNCTIONS	SOURCES	RDA*
Manganese	Structural element of bone and tendon; component of some enzymes	Bran, coffee, tea, nuts, legumes	Adults: 2.5-5.0 mg*
Copper	Involved in storage & release from storage of iron to form hemoglobin	Organ meats, shell-fish, nuts, dried legumes	Adults: 2.0-3.0 mg*
Zinc	Important constituent of enzymes	Meat, fish, eggs, milk	Males 23-50: 15 mg; Females 23-50: 15 mg
Chromium	Necessary for utilization of glucose.	Brewer's yeast, whole grains, liver	Adults: 0.05-0.2 mg*
Selenium	Anti-oxidant (protects & functions with vitamin E)	Depends on soil content where plants are grown and animals are raised	Adults: 0.05-0.2 mg*
Fluorine	Necessary to form and protect teeth; may help retain calcium in bones of elderly	Fluoridated water, seafood, tea	Adults: 1.5-4.0 mg*
Molybdenum	Component of an essential enzyme	Meat, grains, legumes (but content varies greatly according to where grown)	Adults: 0.15-0.5 mg

*Of these elements, an RDA has been established only for zinc; the other values are Estimated Safe and Adequate Daily Dietary Intakes.

PART FOUR
VITAMINS IN FOOD

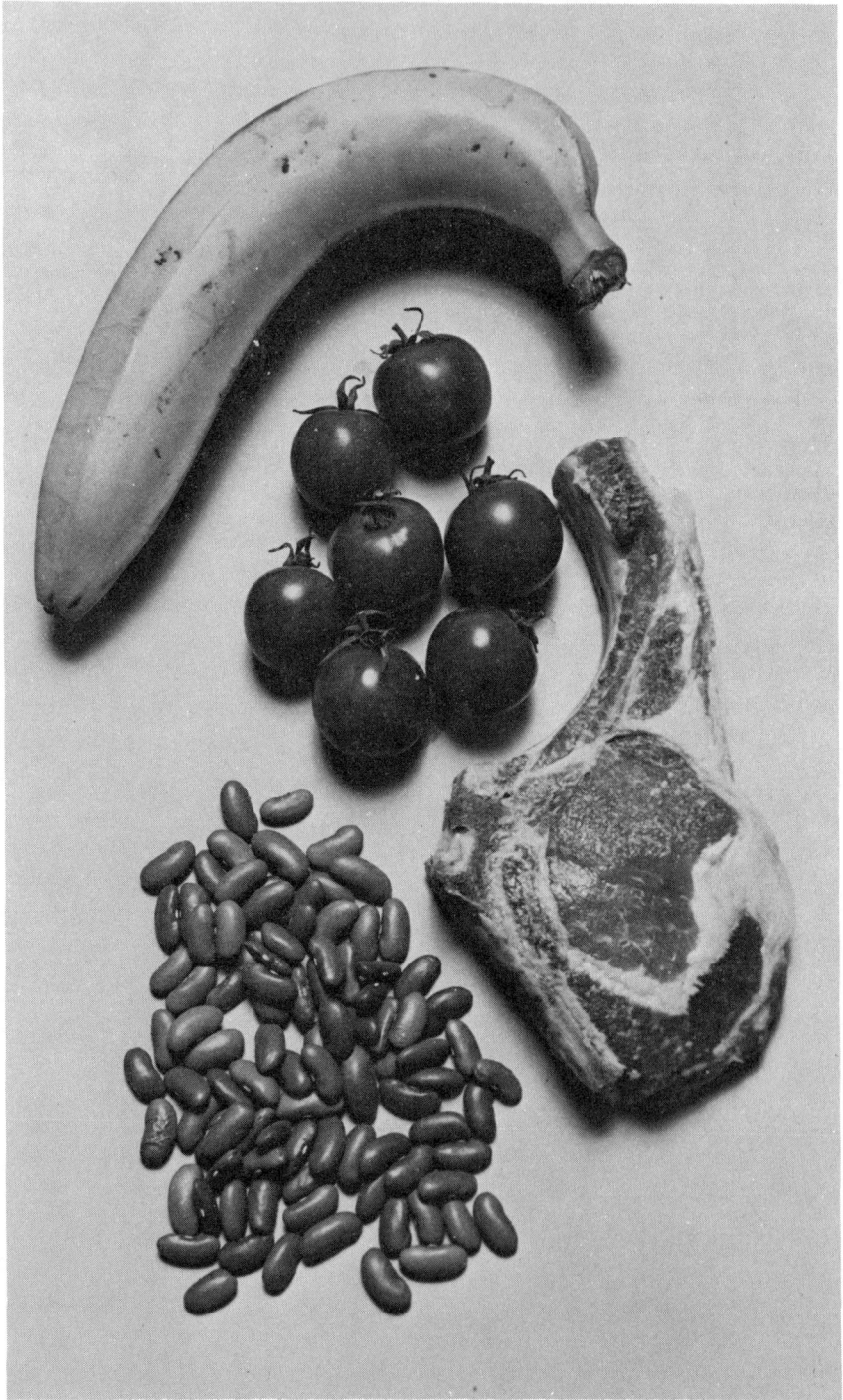

19

Are You Coming Up Short?

ARE YOU COMING UP SHORT?

Because of poor diets, problems with absorption, drug interference or increased demands, some groups are more susceptible than others to lowered levels of vitamins and minerals. Notice we said "lowered levels" and not "deficiencies"; most often such individuals are still well within the safe range for the vitamins in question. Thus, we do not mean to imply that anyone who falls into one of these categories should be taking supplements; indeed, only a small percentage of Americans have problem deficiencies, and these can either be made up with an improvement in diet or are the result of a disorder that requires a doctor's care. If you fall into one of the susceptible groups, it would be a wise idea to examine your diet to see if you are providing for increased needs. Self-diagnosis of disorders and self-prescription of large doses of supplements are not recommended. Pregnant and nursing women, in particular, are advised to consult their physicians before beginning any type of vitamin/mineral supplementation. The same is advised before administering supplements to infants and children. The following is intended as a guide for dietary improvement, but in some cases your physician may wish to prescribe a multivitamin/mineral supplement or a low-dosage individual supplement.

GROUP   **MAY HAVE LOWERED LEVELS OF:**

Group	A	Thiamin	Rib.	Niacin	B6	Folacin
Elderly Women		•	•	•	•	•
Elderly Men		•	•	•	•	•
Pregnant Women*	•	•			•	•
Nursing Women*		•				•
Menstruating Women**						
Infants						
Heavy Drinkers		•		•	•	•
Users of Oral Contraceptives		•	•		•	•
Prolonged Users of Antibiotics		•				
Regular Users of Other Prescription Drugs***	•		•	•	•	•
Chronically Ill						•
Heavy Smokers						
Persons With Disorders That Interfere With Fat Absorption****	•					
Gastrectomy Patients						
Post-operative and Burn Patients						
Vegans						
Fad Dieters and Persons on Strict Low-Calorie Diets *****						
Shut-ins						
Poor		•				
Adolescents						
Children						

GROUP	B12	Biotin	Pan. Acid	C	D	E	K	Calcium	Iron
Elderly Women	•	•	•	•	•			•	
Elderly Men	•	•	•	•	•				
Pregnant Women*	•			•					•
Nursing Women*									•
Menstruating Women**									•
Infants				•		•	•		•
Heavy Drinkers				•					
Users of Oral Contraceptives	•			•					
Prolonged Users of Antibiotics		•	•				•		
Regular Users of Other Prescription Drugs***	•			•	•	•	•		
Chronically Ill				•					
Heavy Smokers				•					
Person With Disorders That Interfere With Fat Absorption****					•	•	•		
Gastrectomy Patients	•								
Post-operative and Burn Patients				•					
Vegans	•								•
Fad Dieters and Persons on Strict Low-Calorie Diets				•					•
Shut-ins					•				
Poor				•					
Adolescents									•
Children									•

    * Doctors often recommend a single multi-vitamin/mineral supplement.
   ** It is nearly impossible for women of child-bearing age to get enough iron in the diet.
  *** See chapter on vitamin/drug interactions.
 **** I.E., cystic fibrosis, cirrhosis, hepatitis, pancreas and gall bladder disease, intestinal disorders, obstructive jaundice.
***** May need multi-vitamin/mineral supplement.

VITAMINS A TO K

VITAMIN	TYPE	GOOD SOURCES	DEFICIENCY
A	oil-soluble	Fish-liver oils, liver, butter, whole milk, cheese, egg yolk, dark green leafy vegetables, yellow-orange vegetables & fruits, fortified products.	Night blindness, eye inflammation, dry, rough skin, reduced resistance to infection, diarrhea. In children: stunted growth, damage to central nervous system.
B1 (THIA-MIN)	water-soluble	Pork, liver & organ meats, brewer's yeast, wheat germ, whole-grain cereals & breads, enriched cereals & breads, soybeans, peanuts & other legumes, milk.	Loss of appetite, nausea, heart problems, muscle contractions, mental confusion, edema, impaired growth, beriberi.
B2 (RIBO-FLAVIN)	water-soluble	Milk, cheese, liver & organ meats, meat, eggs, green leafy vegetables, yeast, enriched foods.	(Linked to other B vitamin deficiencies): cracks at corners of mouth, inflamed, sore lips, inflamed, discolored tongue, dermatitis, anemia, impaired vision, stunted growth.
NIACIN	water-soluble	Lean meat, fish, poultry, liver & organ meats, whole-grain & enriched cereals & breads, green leafy vegetables, peanuts, brewer's yeast.	Indigestion, diarrhea, weight loss, weakness, dermatitis, mental disturbance, pellagra.
B6 (PYRI-DOXINE)	water-soluble	Wheat germ, meat, liver & organ meats, whole-grain cereals, soybeans, peanuts & other legumes, corn.	(Rare) inflamed mouth & tongue, depression, irritability, convulsions, dermatitis, nausea, microcytic anemia, etc.
FOLACIN	water-soluble	Widespread in foods, liver & organ meats, yeast, green leafy vegetables, legumes, whole grains, nuts.	Macrocytic anemia, stunted growth, damage to lining of intestinal tract, impaired resistance to infection.
B12	water-soluble	Animal foods only: liver, meat, fish, poultry, milk, eggs, etc.	Macrocytic anemia, stunted growth, etc.
BIOTIN	water-soluble	Liver, sweetbreads, yeast, eggs, legumes, nuts.	(Extremely rare) inflamed, dry skin, hair loss, lethargy, loss of appetite, etc.

Cont. next page

Cont. from previous page

VITAMINS A TO K

VITAMIN	TYPE	GOOD SOURCES	DEFICIENCY
PANTO-THENIC ACID	water-soluble	Present in most plant & animal tissue: liver & organ meats, yeast, eggs, peanuts & other legumes, wheat germ, whole-grain cereals, beef, vegetables & fruit, salmon, milk.	(Rare) gastrointestinal disturbance, depression, confusion, irritability, insomnia, leg cramps, etc.
C (ASCORBIC ACID)	water-soluble	Citrus fruits, tomatoes, strawberries, melons, broccoli, cauliflower, leafy green vegetables, potatoes, etc.	Easy bruising, bleeding gums, scurvy.
D	oil-soluble	Exposure to sunlight, fish liver oils, fortified milk.	Rickets, osteomalacia (loss of calcium from bones in adults).
E	oil-soluble	Wheat germ & vegetable oils, wheat germ, nuts, legumes, green leafy vegetables, egg yolk, liver.	Unknown in persons eating normal, mixed diet. May cause anemia in premature babies fed inadequate formula.
K	oil-soluble	Green leafy vegetables, cauliflower, liver, egg yolk.	Delayed coagulation of blood, excessive bleeding.

VITAMIN	SIGNS OF OVERDOSE	FUNCTION	RDA (Recommended Daily Amount) MALE 23-50	FEMALE 23-50
A	Headache, nausea, diarrhea, stunted growth, dry, cracked skin, bone pain, loss of appetite, hair loss, menstrual problems, blurred vision, irritability, etc.	Needed for normal vision. Protects against night blindness. Maintains epithelial cells & keeps them resistant to infection.	1000 RE	800 RE
B1 (THIAMIN)	May cause hypersensitivity.	Conversion of food to energy. Conversion of tryptophan to niacin. Component of nerve cell membranes & neurotransmitters.	1.4 mg	1.0 mg

Cont. next page

Cont. from previous page

VITAMIN	SIGNS OF OVERDOSE	FUNCTION	RDA (Recommended Daily Amount)	
			MALE 23-50	FEMALE 23-50
B2 (RIBO-FLAVIN	None currently known.	Conversion of food to energy. Production of red blood cells & hormones.	1.6 mg	1.2 mg
NIACIN	Flushing, sweating, vomiting, diarrhea, skin rash, may reactivate peptic ulcers, irregular heartbeat, loss of appetite, abdominal pain, liver damage, etc.	Conversion of food to energy.	18 mg	13 mg
B6 (PYRI-DOXINE)	Unclear: perhaps sleepiness, B6 dependency.	Component of hemo globin. Metabolism of amino acids. Conversion of tryptophan to niacin, etc.	2.2 mg	2.0 mg
FOLACIN	None currently known; could interfere with diagnosis of pernicious anemia.	Amino acid metabolism. DNA synthesis.	400 mcg	400 mcg
B12	Unclear. Possible nervous system damage if taken orally to correct pernicious anemia.	Metabolism of nutrients. Maintain normal hemoglobin. DNA synthesis. Component of nerve cells.	3.0 mcg	3.0 mcg
BIOTIN	None currently known.	Coenzyme, functions in metabolism of major nutrients.	100-200 mcg*	100-200 mcg*
PANTO-THENIC-ACID	In extremely large doses, diarrhea, water retention.	Necessary for metabolism of major nutrients. Component of sterols, hemoglobin & neurotransmitters.	4-7 mg*	4-7 mg*
C (ASCOR-BIC ACID)	Diarrhea, cramps, kidney stones, C dependency, etc.	Formation & maintenance of collagen. Needed for healthy gums, resistance to infection, wound healing. Amino acid metabolism. Synthesis of hormones & neurotransmitters.	60 mg	60 mg

Cont. next page

Cont. from previous page

RDA
(Recommended Daily Amount)

VITAMIN	SIGNS OF OVERDOSE	FUNCTION	MALE 23-50	FEMALE 23-50
D	Kidney stones, calcification of tissues, nausea, stunted physical & mental growth, stiffness, aches, headache, etc.	Aids calcium absorption. Formation & maintenance of bones & teeth.	5 mcg	5 mcg
E	May produce flu-like symptoms in extremely large doses. May interfere with blood clotting.	Not fully understood. Works as anti-oxidant.	10 mg	8 mg
K	Can cause red blood cells to rupture & release compounds that accumulate in blood & brain, causing serious damage; affects liver's ability to excrete bile.	Aids blood clotting.	70-140 mcg*	70-140 mcg*

*Estimated safe and adequate daily dietary intakes.

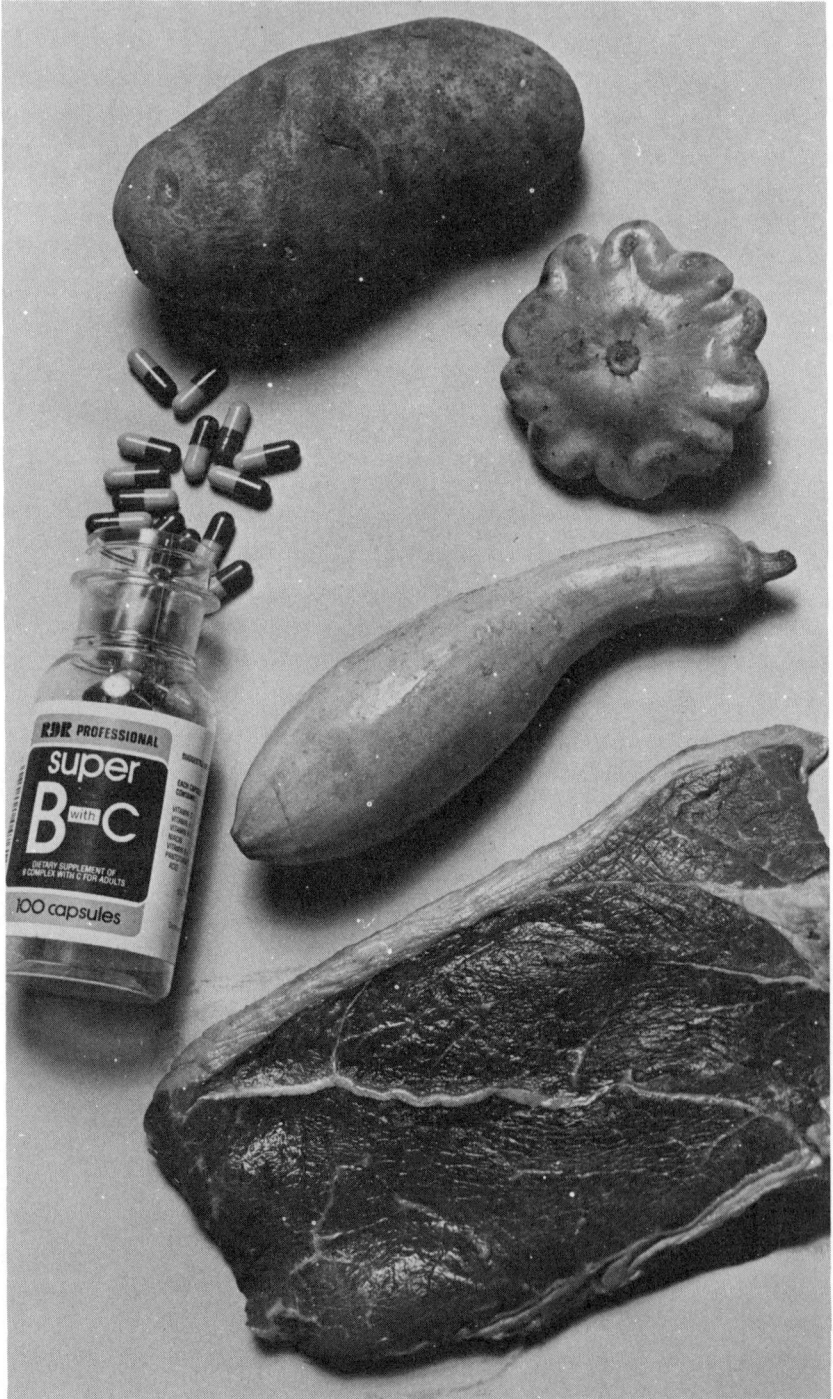

20

Getting Your Vitamins From Food

GETTING YOUR VITAMINS FROM FOOD

One of the most useful tools of the vitamin salesman's trade is the fear most of us have of the food we eat. It's grown on depleted soil with chemical fertilizers, they tell us, and processed to the point that it has all the nutritional value of the flashy packages it comes in. It's certainly true that the foods we eat have changed considerably over the years...and not always for the good. As Jane Brody points out, over half the foods we eat are processed and 50 percent of them didn't even exist as little as ten years ago.

There is genuine cause to be concerned about the nutritional value of many of the foods we consume today. Processed foods provide much greater profit margins than do fresh, whole ones, so the stripping of foods for the sake of greed and convenience is bound not only to continue, but to increase. But that doesn't necessarily mean we have to pay through the nose once to buy nutritionless foods and then pay through the nose again to buy the vitamins and minerals that belong in them. It *is* still possible to obtain the nutrients we need from our foods *if* we choose the right foods and prepare them properly. Unfortunately, it takes just a little extra time and trouble on our part. Fast food restaurants don't fill our street corners—and convenience foods our super-market shelves—for no reason. The fact is that most of us would much rather brown 'n serve, heat 'n eat, and shake 'n pour than take the time to prepare fresh, whole foods. And just as we expect vitamins to make up for smoking or drinking too much or our dozens of other over-indulgences, we expect them to save us from our quick 'n easy but nutritionally empty diets. Sadly, that is not the case. We need more—some forty-odd substances in all—from our food than just vitamins. We can't get everything in pill form, nor do we even know if we have identified all of the essential nutrients. The best health insurance is still the proper selection and preparation of foods. Let the following tips be your guide and if you are a normal, healthy individual, you should never find yourself in need of vitamin supplements.

GO FOR THE NATURAL

Natural food isn't something you buy in a health food store and rarely does it have the word "natural" anywhere on the label....when it has a label. It is simply the fresh, whole food you can buy at any grocery store, meat and fish market or produce stand. Going for the natural means passing up already prepared convenience foods, quick mixes and tasty treats comprised of sugar, salt, white flour, and artificial colors and flavors, in favor of fresh meats, fish, poultry, and produce, whole-grain breads and cereals, nuts, legumes, and dairy products.

Going for the natural also means understanding the wide scope of the word "processing." To most of us that word has totally negative connotations, but it is important to remember that processing can simply mean cutting, cooking or freezing a food. While some foods are processed for the sake of profit and convenience, many more are processed to keep them in a safe and nutritious form for as long as possible to assure an adequate and varied food supply year round. Thus, while freshly picked food is always the ultimate to be striven for, canned and frozen foods (i.e., vegetables, meats, etc.) are also a wholesome and necessary part of the diet. In fact, a food that is picked ripe and canned or frozen immediately is very often a better nutritional buy than a "fresh" product that is picked green and has seen several days of transport and several more setting on a produce counter. If you have a choice between frozen or canned, choose frozen since fruits and vegetables lose many of their water-soluble vitamins to the water and high heat of canning.

CHOOSE A VARIETY

Getting stuck in monotonous food consumption patterns is poor nutrition, no matter how "healthy" the few foods you choose to eat. Most foods contain more than one nutrient, but no food supplies everything you need. The best way to get those forty-odd nutrients—plus any we may not know about yet—is to eat a wide variety of foods that we know have a good distribution of a number of the nutrients we know something about. In that way, you should be getting at least adequate amounts of the less understood ones, as well. Selecting a broad array of foods protects you in other ways, too.

Remember that problem of depleted soil we mentioned earlier? First of all, it must be said that it isn't quite the problem vitamin vendors would have us believe. Plants need many of the same nutrients we need; without those nutrients the plants will not grow. In answer to the question of whether our soil is depleted, nutritionist Ronald M. Deutsch has said, "In that case, the plant simply won't grow. If the soil is just poorish, the plant may grow, but be stunted and fewer plants will grow on an acre. But each plant that does grow *has* to be nutritionally complete. Endless analyses by state and federal agricultural laboratories show that each ounce of each potato, bean, etc., is the nutritive equivalent of every other ounce of the same variety." Soil fertility has not been shown to be a determining factor in the level of vitamins in crops. Plants that grow normally and produce satisfactory yields can be expected to contain vitamins characteristic of their species and variety.

As for the use of chemical fertilizers, according to the Committee on Nutritional Misinformation of the National Academy of Sciences, "No laboratory test or animal feeding study has been developed that distinguishes crops grown with inorganic from those grown with organic fertilizers. There also is no reliable evidence that organic fertilizers are a better means of providing essential elements for plants and in turn for man than are inorganic fertilizers." It is also true, however, that commercial farms that use inorganic fertilizers also usually return large quantities of organic materials to the soil, so organic fertilization is actually a part of most farming in the U.S. anyway.

There are some nutrients that have been depleted from the soil in some regions....or simply did not exist there to begin with. The plants grown on these lands continue to thrive because, unlike people, they do not happen to need these particular nutrients. Iodine is a notable example. Plants don't need it, people do. If it is in the soil it will be in the plants grown on that soil, but if it isn't it won't and the plants will be normal and healthy. That's why, earlier in this century, when people ate primarily what was grown in their own region, we developed what was known as the goiter belt across the central U.S., goiter being, of course, the iodine deficiency disease. Today the problem has largely been controlled by the use of iodized salt. However, the reality of a nutritional deficiency developing in that way is an excellent advertisement for the wisdom of eating a wide variety of foods.

In this day of rapid transportation, the counters in our supermarkets contain a wide variety of fresh, frozen, canned and packaged foods from all over the country and the world. Eating a broad array of them should be pretty good insurance that you are getting foods grown on a variety of soils of varying nutrient contents. It also reduces the likelihood of being exposed to excessive amounts of contaminants in any one food. Just as toxicants can occur in foods as the result of processing or pesticide use, many occur naturally in some foods and others occur naturally in the soil on which foods are grown (i.e., the food grown in some regions has exceptionally high levels of the mineral selenium that may be toxic with prolonged consumption). Thus, choosing a wide variety of foods lets you get enough of what you want without getting too much of what you don't.

For some time nutritionists have preached the "Basic Four Food Groups" as the ideal guide to a well-balanced daily diet. The Basic Four recommends daily choices from the following groups: Milk, Meat, Fruit and Vegetable, and Cereal. While the Basic Four has served us well in virtually eliminating deficiency diseases from this country, it has, because of its emphasis on high-fat foods, put us on a collision course with heart disease, cancer, stroke, etc. In an excellent new book entitled *Jack Sprat's Legacy: The Science and Politics of Fat & Cholesterol*, Patricia Hausman of the Center For Science In the Public Interest says:

"By the 1960s (nutritionists) could not help but conclude that the Basic Four was not serving us well enough. American men, despite their diet rich in protein, vitamins and minerals, were about six times as likely to die of heart attacks as Japanese men. Rates of certain cancers also differed dramatically between the two countries; colon and breast cancers were five times as common in the United States. Researchers realized that pollution, smoking, and hectic lifestyles were not the likely explanation; the United States and Japan had all three in common. Study after study implicated diet as an important explanation for the differences. The most outstanding difference between the Japanese and American diets was the fat content; Americans were eating two to four times as much fat as the Japanese. The message was that some of the nutritionists' most revered foods were not so flawless after all. Despite their nutrient value, egg yolk, and certain meat and dairy products are high in fat or cholesterol, a fat-like substance also linked to heart disease."

Hausman concludes, however, that the Basic Four can be salvaged, and gives prescriptions for each group. The book is recommended reading for anyone genuinely concerned about the real health problems that face us in the latter half of the 20th century. Meanwhile, to alter the Basic Four to a still very useful guide, it is only necessary to trim the fat out of it. Remember, for example, that the Milk Group contains not only whole milk and ice cream, but a wide variety of low-fat and non-fat milks, yogurts and cheeses, and that the Meat Group contains, in addition to red meat, poultry, fish, legumes and grain protein. We also need to forget the myth that starches are fattening and place more emphasis on the Fruit and Vegetable and Cereal (preferably whole grain) Groups.

Currently, the American diet contains approximately 42 percent of calories from fat. To radically improve our diet we would be wise to try to get that down to under 30 percent. Fifteen percent of calories should then come from protein and 55 percent from carbohydrates, preferably the complex kind found in fruits, vegetables and whole grains.

BASIC FOUR FOOD GROUPS

MILK GROUP—*Adults/two servings; teenagers/four servings, children/three servings.* Includes: Milk—whole, low-fat, non-fat, evaporated, dry; buttermilk; cheese (regular and low-fat); cottage cheese; ice cream and ice milk; yogurt, etc.

MEAT GROUP—*Two servings.* Includes: Beef; veal; lamb; pork; fish; poultry; eggs; dry beans; dry peas; lentils; nuts; peanuts and peanut butter; soybeans; and grain protein.

VEGETABLE-FRUIT GROUP—*Four servings.*

BREAD-CEREAL GROUP—(Whole-grain and enriched products are recommended). Includes: Bread; cooked and ready-to-eat cereals; cornmeal; crackers; flour; grits; macaroni, spaghetti and noodles; rice; baked goods.

Milk Group

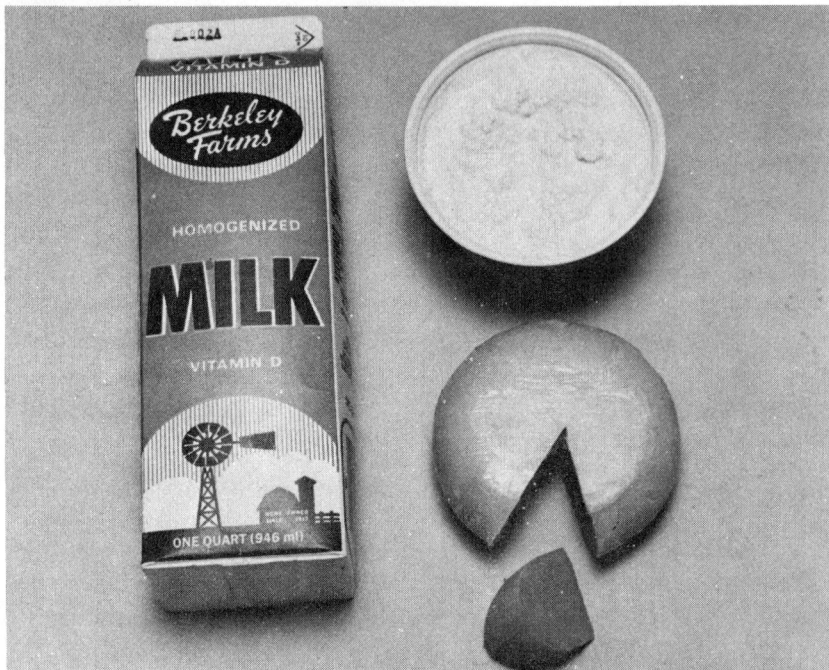

Meat Group

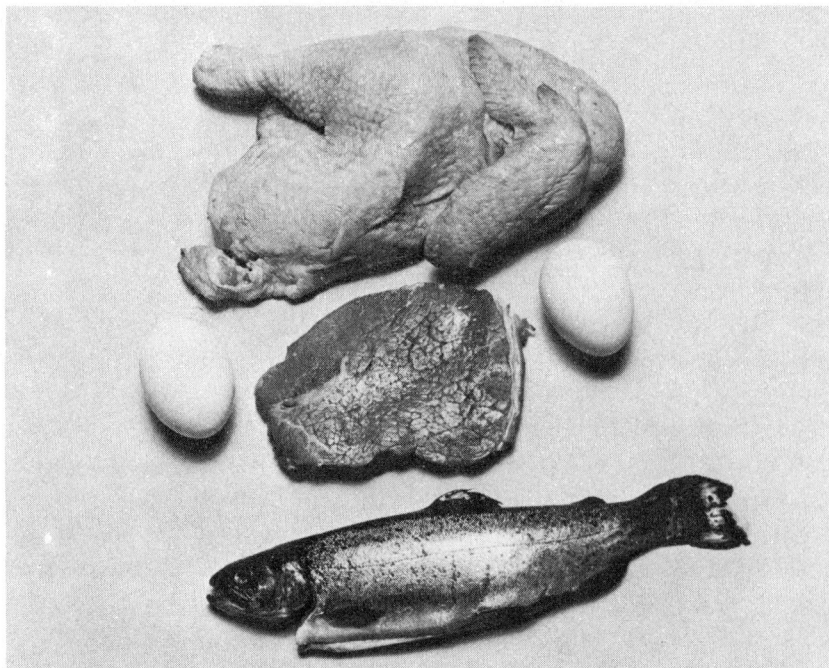

Vegetable Group

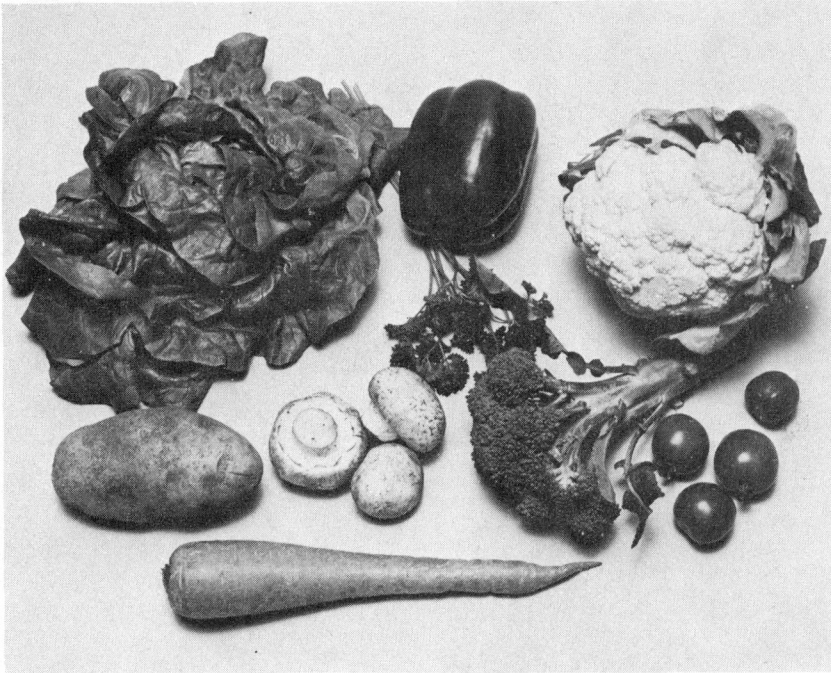

Fruit Group

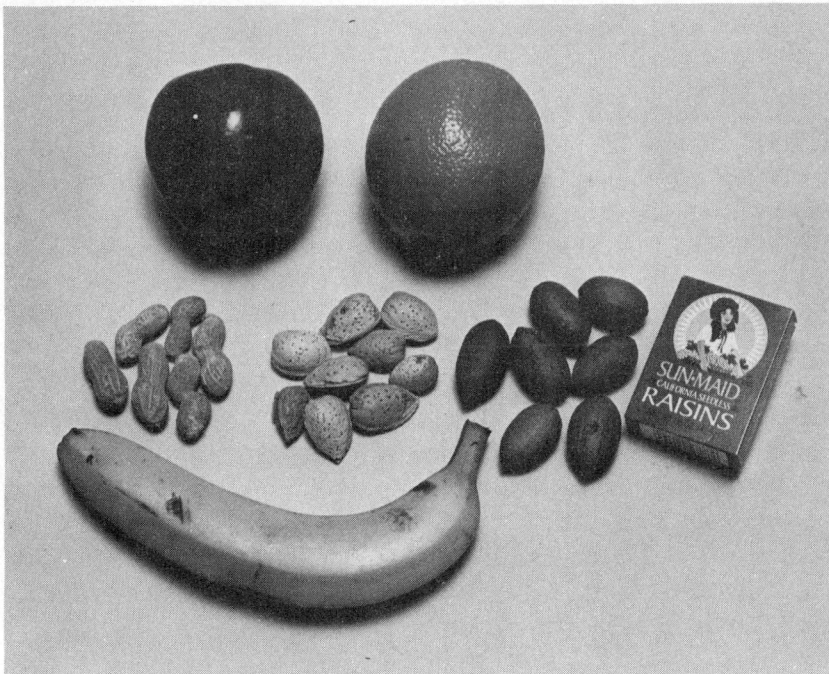

Bread-Cereal Group

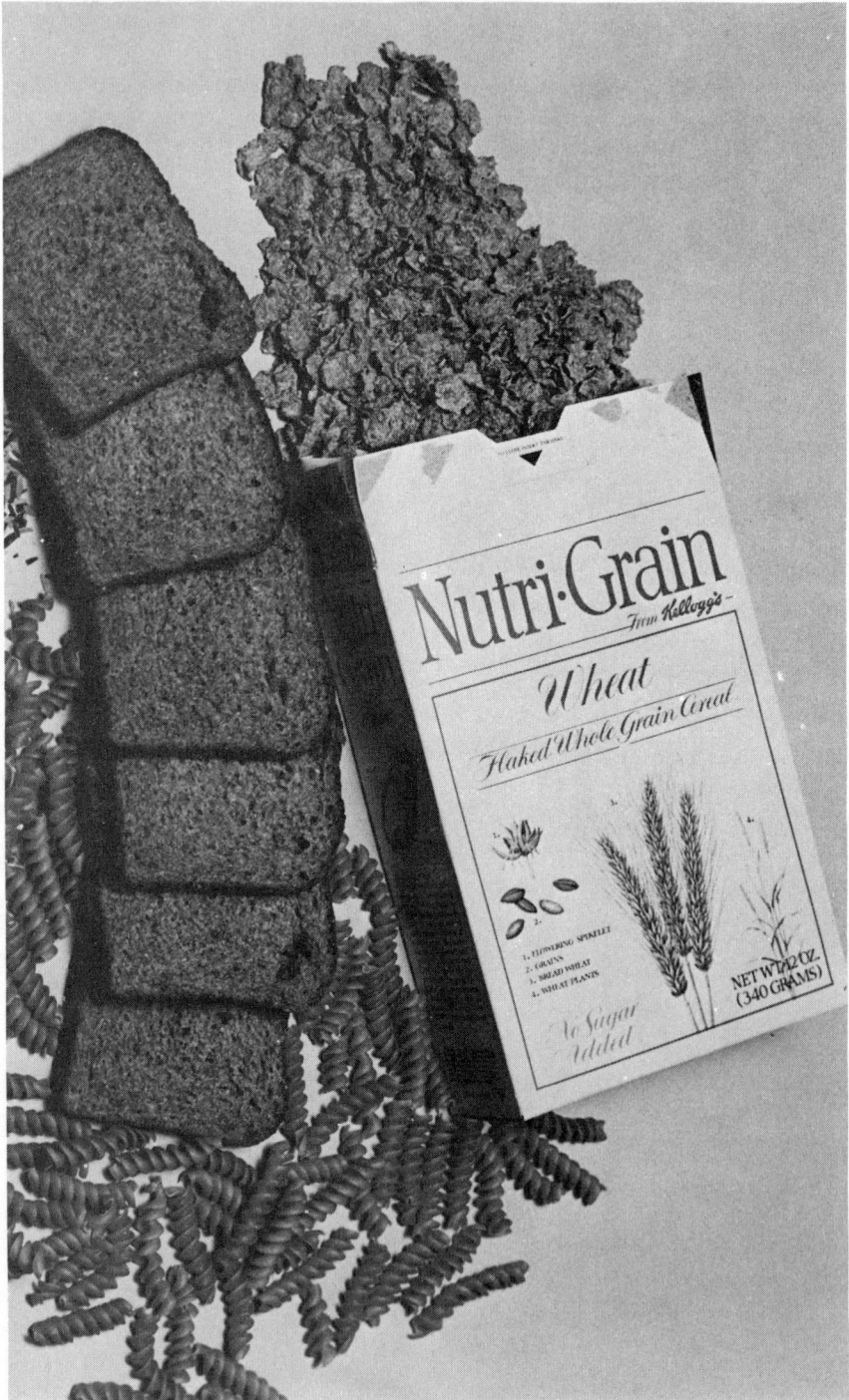

BUY FRESH, STORE PROPERLY, USE PROMPTLY, AND COOK CAREFULLY

Foods, particularly fresh fruits and vegetables, quickly lose their vitamins with age. To make sure you are getting your money's worth nutritionally, buy the freshest foods you can find and store them properly for as short a time as possible. Many of the following tips come from the USDA publications "Conserving The Nutritive Values In Foods" and "Family Fare: A Guide To Good Nutrition." (Both publications, as well as "How To Buy Fresh Fruits" and "How To Buy Fresh Vegetables," are available from the U.S. Government Printing Office, Washington, D.C. 20402).

BUYING

- Buy eggs that are kept in refrigerated cases.

- Buy fruits and vegetables that do not show signs of aging (i.e., firm fruits without bruises or soft spots; lettuce that is green, crisp and firm; broccoli without yellowing, soft or spreading heads, etc.).

- Try to buy only as much produce at one time as you can use in a day or two; significant vitamin loss occurs with prolonged storage at home.

- Buy vine- or tree-ripened fruits and vegetables whenever possible.

- Deep orange carrots and sweet potatoes have much more vitamin A value than paler ones.

- Dark green, leafy vegetables are richer in nutrients than light green ones.

- When buying frozen foods, select packages that are frozen solid. Avoid partially thawed packages that feel soft or are stained, indications of thawing and refreezing.

- Pay attention to open dating on food containers; buy those with the most distant expiration dates.

STORING

- Store milk in a covered, opaque container and keep it cold. Calcium, protein and vitamin A are relatively stable in milk, but the high riboflavin content can be reduced or destroyed by improper handling.

- Contrary to popular belief, frozen and canned foods continue to lose their nutrients. Even if, as recommended, your freezer is kept at 0 degrees F or below, nutrients—particularly vitamin C— will be lost with time. If you have a large freezer, date foods. Use frozen foods as rapidly as possible to assure optimal nutrition. "Family Fare" suggests that frozen foods can be stored in the freezing unit of a refrigerator up to one week; for longer storage foods should be kept in a freezer at 0 degrees. Do not thaw and refreeze.

● Keep canned foods in a cool (70 degrees or below), dry place and limit the length of storage. The longer the storage period and the higher the temperature, the greater the loss of nutrients. If canned foods are stored at 65 degrees, only about 10 percent of vitamin C is lost in a year; when the temperature is 80 degrees, losses may reach 25 percent. Carotene or provitamin A losses average only about 10 percent in a year when cans are stored at 80 degrees. Thiamin in canned fruits and vegetables is well-retained when stored for one year at 65 degrees. When stored at 80 degrees for one year, losses may increase to 15 percent in canned fruits and to 25 percent in canned vegetables. Canned meats can lose their thiamin content in storage. For example, pork may lose up to 20 percent of its thiamin by the end of three months and 30 percent in six months at 70 degrees. Higher temperatures mean greater losses.

● Store dried fruits in tightly closed containers at room temperature (not above 70 degrees F). In warm, humid weather, refrigerate.

● Refrigerate lard, butter, margarine, salad dressing, drippings and opened containers of cooking and salad oils. Most firm vegetable shortenings can be stored covered at room temperature.

● Store eggs in the refrigerator, large end up.

● Remove meats and fish from butcher paper and rewrap or store in covered container for up to three to five days.

● Storing cooked vegetables greatly diminishes their vitamin content. You may save time by cooking large quantities ahead, but you lose some nutrients.

● Store fruits and vegetables according to the following chart:

STORAGE GUIDE FOR FRUITS & VEGETABLES

Hold at room temperature until ripe; then refrigerate, uncovered: apples, apricots, avocados, berries (do not wash before refrigerating), cherries, melons (except watermelons), nectarines, peaches, pears, plums, tomatoes (do not ripen in the sun or in the refrigerator).

Store in cool room or refrigerate, uncovered: grapefruit, lemons, limes, oranges.

Store in cool room, away from bright light: onions—mature, potatoes, rutabagas, squash—winter, sweet potatoes.

Refrigerate, covered: asparagus, beans—snap or wax, beets, broccoli, cabbage, carrots, cauliflower, celery, corn—husked, cucumbers, greens, onions—green, parsnips, peas—shelled, peppers—green, radishes, squash—summer, turnips.

Refrigerate, uncovered: beans, lima—in pods, corn—in husks, grapes, peas—in pods, pineapples, watermelons.

Source: "Family Fare: A Guide To Good Nutrition."

PREPARATION

Foods differ greatly in nutrient content and nutrients vary greatly in their stability. While some nutrients are very stable, others are destroyed to varying degrees by such things as heat, light, exposure to oxygen, etc. Thus, the best type of preparation for maximum nutrient conservation will vary from one food to another; following are some good general tips, however, for keeping nutrients in cooked foods.

● Do not chop vegetables and fruits any smaller than necessary.

● Clean, chop and cook vegetables as close to meal time as possible.

● When cleaning vegetables, don't throw out the most nutritious parts. For example, the leafy parts of collard greens, turnip greens and kale have more vitamin A value than the stems or midribs. The outer, green leaves of lettuce, while perhaps not as appealing as the tender inner leaves, have more calcium, iron and vitamin A. The core of cabbage, like the leaves, is high in vitamin C. Broccoli leaves have more vitamin A than the stalks or flower buds and are very tasty, yet many of us discard these.

● A very sharp blade is recommended when cutting or trimming vegetables as they lose vitamins A and C when bruised.

● Cook vegetables only until tender. Keep cooking of all foods to a minimum.

● Use as little water as possible in cleaning and cooking. Retain cooking water for use in soups, sauces, gravies, etc. The less water you cook in and throw away, the more water-soluble vitamins you retain.

● Cook food covered whenever possible, using tight-fitting lids.

● Add vegetables to boiling water rather than bringing the water to a boil with the vegetables soaking.

● Boiling or baking potatoes, carrots, sweet potatoes, etc. whole and in their skins retains nearly all their nutrients. When cut and peeled, losses are significant.

● Do not allow food to stand exposed to heat, light and air.

● Cooking in iron vessels is a good way to get extra amounts of that mineral in the diet.

● After canning, the water-soluble nutrients in vegetables distribute themselves evenly throughout the solids and liquid. Serve the liquid along with canned vegetables or use it in soup, etc.

● Meat drippings that result from thawing, cooking and slicing contain some of the B vitamins. After the fat is skimmed off, drippings can be used in soups, gravies, etc.

● Cooking beef to the rare stage conserves more thiamin than cooking it to the well-done stage.

● Cooking cereals (i.e., pasta, rice, etc.) in large quantities of water and rinsing afterward costs you nutrients.

● Packaged rice has already been cleaned. Washing it before cooking can cause a thiamin loss of 25 percent in regular white rice and 10 percent in brown or parboiled rice.

● To preserve thiamin in baking, follow these steps: bake only until crust is light brown; limit the surface area exposed to heat (i.e., less thiamin is lost baking cornbread than corn sticks); toast bread only lightly and use thicker slices for toasting.

PART FIVE
LABELS, ALCOHOL AND PICKING PILLS

PASTEURIZED
VIT A & D
NONFAT MILK

NUTRITION INFORMATION PER SERVING

SERVING SIZE.......................... ONE CUP
SERVINGS PER CONTAINER......... 4
CALORIES 90
PROTEIN............................ 9 GRAMS
CARBOHYDRATE.................... 12 GRAMS
FAT................................. 0 GRAMS

PERCENTAGE OF U.S. RECOMMENDED
DAILY ALLOWANCES (U.S. RDA)

PROTEIN	20	VITAMIN D	25
VITAMIN A	10	VITAMIN B_6	4
VITAMIN C	4	VITAMIN B_{12}	15
THIAMINE	8	PHOSPHORUS ...	25
RIBOFLAVIN	30	MAGNESIUM	10
NIACIN	*	ZINC	6
CALCIUM	30	PANTOTHENIC	
IRON	*	ACID	6

*CONTAINS LESS THAN 2% OF THE
U.S. RDA OF THESE NUTRIENTS

NONFAT MILK WITH NONFAT MILK
SOLIDS, VITAMIN A PALMITATE
AND VITAMIN D_3 ADDED

DIST. BY SAFEWAY STORES, INC.
HEAD OFFICE, OAKLAND, CA. 94660
PROCESSED AND FILLED AT LOCATION CODED ABOVE

21

Reading Nutrition Labels

Avid cereal box readers will remember the MDRs (Minimum Daily Requirements) that used to appear on labels of selected foods. The figures represented the percentage contained in the food of the minimum amount of a vitamin or mineral considered necessary to maintain health. The MDRs are now obsolete, replaced by the U.S. RDAs. Because it is impossible to state the minimum amount of a nutrient every individual in America requires, the U.S. RDAs are based on the RDAs and include a generous excess above minimum needs to allow for individual variations.

Because it would be cumbersome to print the entire RDA chart for seventeen separate population groups on package labels, nutrient values are listed as percentages of U.S. RDAs and represent the groups with the highest requirements. For example, the highest requirement for thiamin is among males aged 19 to 22, so it is their requirement for 1.5 mg that becomes the U.S. RDA for thiamin for all adults and children over four years of age. Thus, the U.S. RDA is higher than necessary for all other age groups, but at least all age groups are safely covered.

While most of us are familiar with the U.S. RDA for adults and children four or more years of age, which is the one used on the majority of food and vitamin labels, there are actually four groupings of U.S. RDAs. One of the groups is for infants up to one year and another is for children under four years of age. These are used primarily for labeling baby foods, infant formulas and vitamin supplements intended for these age groups. The fourth category is for pregnant and lactating women and is for use on special dietary foods.

Developed by the Food and Drug Administration, U.S. RDAs are required for nutrition labeling only on foods to which a nutrient has been added, or for which a nutritional claim is made. Many manufacturers print nutritional information even though it is not required. Following is labeling information that should be of interest to nutrition-conscious shoppers.

NUTRITION INFORMATION: Nutrition labels are rquired to give very specific information for each serving of the food or supplement in question. First they tell the serving size (for example, "serving size=1 cup"), the number of servings in the container, the number of calories per serving, and the amounts in grams of protein, carbohydrate, and fat per serving. They then tell the percentage of the U.S. RDA of protein and seven specified vitamins and minerals in each serving. These vitamins and minerals and the order in which they must be listed are: vitamin A, vitamin C, thiamin, riboflavin, niacin, calcium and iron. Other essential vitamins and minerals may be listed if the food contains at least two percent of the U.S. RDA per serving, but listing of these nutrients is optional. However, if any specific claim is made on the label (i.e., that the product is low in sodium), the quantitative information is required on the nutrition lable. Following are sample labels from food and vitamin products:

FOOD LABEL

NUTRITION INFORMATION PER SERVING

Serving Size	6 fl. oz. (177 ml)
Servings Per Container	4
Calories	35
Protein	1 Gram
Carbohydrate	8 Grams
Fat	0 Grams

PERCENTAGE OF U.S. RECOMMENDED DAILY ALLOWANCES (U.S. RDA)

Protein	2	Riboflavin	2
Vitamin A	25	Niacin	4
Vitamin C	45	Calcium	*
Thiamin	2	Iron	2

*Contains less than 2 percent of the U.S. RDA of this nutrient.

VITAMIN SUPPLEMENT LABEL

ONE TABLET DAILY SUPPLIES:

Vitamin	Quantity	% of U.S. RDA
Vitamin A	5,000 I.U.	100
Vitamin E	15 I.U.	50
Vitamin C	60 mg	100
Folic Acid	0.4 mg	100
Thiamin	1.5 mg	100
Riboflavin	1.7 mg	100
Niacin	20 mg	100
Vitamin B-6	2 mg	100
Vitamin B-12	6 mcg	100
Vitamin D	400 I.U.	100
Pantothenic Acid	10 mg	100

Minerals	Quantity	% of U.S. RDA
Iron	18 mg	100
Calcium	100 mg	10
Phosphorus	100 mg	10
Iodine	150 mcg	100
Magnesium	100 mg	25
Copper	2 mg	100
Zinc	15 mg	100

LIST OF INGREDIENTS: According to FDA regulations, the ingredients must be listed on most foods. The main ingredient, that is, the one that accounts for the largest part of the product's weight, must be listed first, followed in descending order by the other ingredients. Additives must be listed on the label, but colors and flavors do not have to be listed by name.

ADDED NUTRIENTS: In these days of over-processing, many

foods would have little nutritional value unless vitamins and minerals were added. Foods with added nutrients fall into one of three categories:

Restored — Micronutrients (vitamins and minerals) are added back at the same level as in the food before processing.

Enriched — Vitamins and minerals that occurred naturally in the food are added back, but at a higher level than in the original.

Fortified — Both the nutrients that naturally occurred in the food, plus others that did not, are added to the food.

CLAIMS: We all know the kinds of claims made for certain vitamins and so-called health foods. But if you want to find out just how much faith the manufacturer has that his product can actually accomplish those lofty goals, look on the package. Chances are you will find no claims whatsoever as to what the product can accomplish, because if the label on a food or vitamin product makes false or misleading claims, the FDA can take action on the grounds that the product is mislabeled or misbranded. That still gives quacks and shysters a lot of leeway in the media, but if false claims are made in ads or in other material directly promoting the product, the Federal Trade Commission can take action. But, according to the FDA, consumers still must be wary because, "the labels on or promotions for fad foods or diets often do not make any direct claims that can be shown to be false. Instead, they refer to a book, a pamphlet, a speech, or a magazine article that has praised the product. Thus, these indirect promotions receive the protection of the First Amendment." If it is not directly connected with product promotion, there just is no law that prevents spreading false and even dangerous nutritional information.

U.S. RECOMMENDED DAILY ALLOWANCES (U.S. RDAs)

Vitamins, Minerals and Protein	Unit of Measurement	Infants	Adults and Children 4 or More Years of Age	Children Under 4 Years of Age	Pregnant or Lactating Women
*Vitamin A	International Units	1,500	5,000	2,500	8,000
Vitamin D	,,	400	400[a]	400	400
Vitamin E	,,	5.0	30	10	30
*Vitamin C	Milligrams	35	60	40	60
Folic Acid	,,	0.1	0.4	0.2	0.8
*Thiamine	,,	0.5	1.5	0.7	1.7
*Riboflavin	,,	0.6	1.7	0.8	2.0
*Niacin	,,	8.0	20	9.0	20
Vitamin B-6	,,	0.4	2.0	0.7	2.5
Vitamin B-12	Micrograms	2.0	6.0	3.0	8.0
Biotin	Milligrams	0.5	0.3	0.15	0.3
Pantothenic Acid	,,	3.0	10	5.0	10
*Calcium	Grams	0.6	1.0	0.8	1.3
Phosphorus	,,	0.5	1.0	0.8	1.3
Iodine	Micrograms	45	150	70	150
*Iron	,,	15	18	10	18
Magnesium	,,	70	400	200	450
Copper	,,	0.6	2.0	1.0	2.0
Zinc	,,	5.0	15	8.0	15

*Values of these nutrients must be declared on package labels. Listing of other vitamins and minerals is optional.
Source: Food and Drug Administration.

VITAMIN/MINERAL CONTENT OF SOME COMMON FOODS

FOOD	A	THIA-MIN	RIBO-FLA-VIN	*NIA-CIN	C	CAL-CIUM	IRON
	IU	mg	mg	mg	mg	mg	mg
Meat Group							
Liver (calf, fried, 3 oz.)	27,800	.20	3.54	14	31	11	12.1
Ground beef, lean with 10% fat (broiled, well done, 1 3-oz. patty)	20	.08	.20	5.1	----	10	3.0
Pork loin chops (broiled, 2.7 oz.)	0	.75	.22	4.5	----	9	2.7
T-bone steak, lean, trimmed of separable fat (broiled, 5.8 oz.)	30	.13	.38	9.7	----	20	6.1
Chicken (fried, ½ breast and 1 drumstick)	120	.07	.32	14.3	----	15	2.2
Eggs (scrambled, 2 large)	1,380	.10	.36	trace	0	102	2.2
Tuna, canned in oil, drained (3 oz.)	70	.04	.10	10.1	----	7	1.6
Halibut (broiled w/butter, 1 fillet or 1 steak)	850	.06	.09	10.4	----	20	1.0
Peas, split, dry (cooked, 1 cup)	100	.37	.22	2.2	----	28	4.2
Lima beans (cooked, drained, 1 cup)	----	.25	.11	1.3	----	55	5.9
Peanut butter (1 tbsp.)	----	.02	.02	2.4	0	9	0.3
Cashews (roasted, ¼ cup)	35	.15	.09	0.6	----	13	1.3
Milk Group							
Milk (1 cup)							
whole	350	.07	.41	0.2	2	288	0.1
non-fat	10	.09	.44	0.2	2	296	0.1
low-fat	200	.10	.52	0.2	2	352	0.1
Cheddar cheese (1 oz.)	370	.01	.13	trace	0	213	0.3
Cottage cheese, small or large curd, creamed (1 cup)	420	.07	.61	0.2	0	230	0.7

VITAMIN/MINERAL CONTENT OF SOME COMMON FOODS   CONT.)

FOOD	A	THIA-MIN	RIBO-FLA-VIN	*NIA-CIN	C	CAL-CIUM	IRON
our cream (1 tbsp.)	100	trace	.02	trace	trace	12	trace
ogurt, made from par- ally skimmed milk	170	.10	.44	0.2	2	294	0.1
e cream (1 cup)	590	.05	.28	0.1	1	194	0.1
e milk (1 cup)	280	.07	.29	0.1	1	204	0.1
egetable Group (fresh)							
sparagus (cooked, drained, spears)	540	.10	.11	0.8	16	13	0.4
reen beans (cooked, drained, cup)	680	.09	.11	0.6	15	63	0.8
roccoli (cooked, drained, cup)	3,880	.14	.31	1.2	140	136	1.2
abbage (raw, finely shredded, cup)	120	.05	.05	0.3	42	44	0.4
arrots (raw, 1 whole)	5,500	.03	.03	0.3	4	18	0.4
ceberg lettuce (¼ head)	375	.07	.07	0.3	7	23	0.6
otatoes							
(baked, peeled after baking, 1 medium)	trace	.10	.04	1.7	20	9	0.7
(french fried, 10 pieces)	trace	.07	.04	1.8	12	9	0.7
(mashed, milk & but- ter added, 1 cup)	330	.16	.10	1.9	18	47	0.8
pinach							
(raw, chopped, 1 cup)	4,460	.06	.11	0.3	28	51	1.7
(cooked, 1 cup)	14,580	.13	.25	1.0	50	167	4.0
weet potatoes (baked, eeled after baking, 1 medium)	8,910	.10	.07	0.7	24	44	1.0
Tomatoes (raw, 3-in. dia- meter, 1)	1,640	.11	.07	1.3	42	24	0.9

VITAMIN/MINERAL CONTENT OF SOME COMMON FOODS   (CONT.)

FOOD	A	THIA-MIN	RIBO-FLA-VIN	*NIA-CIN	C	CAL-CIUM	IRON
Tomato juice (canned, 1 6-oz. glass)	1,460	.09	.05	1.5	29	13	1.6
Turnip greens (cooked, 1 cup)	8,270	.15	.33	0.7	68	252	1.5
Fruit Group (fresh)							
Apple	50	.04	.02	0.1	3	8	0.4
Apricots (3)	2,890	.03	.04	0.7	10	18	0.5
Avocado, California (raw, ½)	315	.12	.22	1.8	15	11	0.7
Banana	230	.06	.07	0.8	12	10	0.8
Cantaloupe (½ medium)	6,540	.08	.06	1.2	63	27	0.8
Orange	260	.13	.05	0.5	66	54	0.5
Orange juice (frozen concentrate, 1 cup)	550	.22	.02	1.0	120	25	0.2
Peach (1 medium)	1,320	.02	.05	1.0	7	9	0.5
Strawberries (1 cup)	90	.04	.10	1.0	88	31	1.5
Bread-Cereal Group							
Bread							
(white, enriched, 2 slices)	trace	.12	.10	1.2	trace	42	1.2
(whole-wheat, 2 slices)	trace	.18	.06	1.6	trace	48	1.6
(rye, 2 slices)	0	.10	.04	0.8	0	38	0.8
Devil's food cake w/chocolate icing (1 piece)	100	.02	.06	0.2	trace	41	0.6
Chocolate chip cookies (3)	30	.03	.03	0.3	trace	12	0.6
Corn muffin, enriched (1)	120	.08	.09	0.6	trace	42	0.7
Saltine crackers (4)	0	trace	trace	0.1	0	2	0.1
Macaroni (cooked, 1 cup)							
(enriched)	0	.20	.11	1.5	0	8	1.3
(unenriched)	0	.01	.01	0.4	0	11	0.6
Oatmeal (cooked, 1 cup)	0	.19	.05	0.2	0	22	1.4
Pizza, cheese (1/8 of 14-in. diameter pie)	290	.04	.12	0.7	4	107	0.7

VITAMIN/MINERAL CONTENT OF SOME COMMON FOODS   (CONT.)

FOOD	A	THIA-MIN	RIBO-FLA-VIN	*NIA-CIN	C	CAL-CIUM	IRON
Rice (cooked, 1 cup)							
(white, enriched)	0	.23	.02	2.1	0	21	1.8
(white, unenriched)	0	.04	.02	0.8	0	21	0.4
(brown, long grain)	0	.18	.04	2.7	0	23	1.0
Bran flakes w/raisins, added thiamin & iron	trace	.16	.07	2.7	0	28	13.5

Miscellaneous

FOOD	A	THIA-MIN	RIBO-FLA-VIN	*NIA-CIN	C	CAL-CIUM	IRON
Butter (1 pat)	170	----	----	----	0	1	0
Margarine (1 pat)	170	----	----	----	0	1	0
Oil, corn (1 tbsp.)	----	0	0	0	0	0	0
Mayonnaise (1 tbsp.)	40	trace	.01	trace	----	3	0.1
Blue cheese dressing (1 tbsp.)	30	trace	.02	trace	trace	12	trace
Honey (1 tbsp.)	0	trace	.01	.1	trace	1	0.1
Beer (12 fl. oz.)	----	.01	.11	2.2	----	18	trace
Liquor, 80 proof (1½ fl. oz.)	----	----	----	----	----	----	----
Wine (3½ fl. oz.)	----	trace	.01	0.1	----	9	0.4
Olives (3 small)	10	trace	trace	----	----	9	0.1
White sauce (½ cup)	575	.05	.22	0.3	1	144	0.3
Cola (12 fl. oz.)	0	0	0	0	0	----	----

*   Represents preformed niacin only, not tryptophan content.

----   Denotes lack of reliable data for a constituent believed to be present in a measurable amount.

Source: Catherine F. Adams, *Nutritive Value of American Foods* (Agriculture Handbook No. 456), (Washington, D.C.: United States Department of Agriculture, 1975), and *Nutritive Value of Foods* (Home and Garden Bulletin No. 72), (Washington, D.C.: USDA, 1971). Both publications may be purchased from Superintendent of Documents, U.S. Government Printing Office, Washington, D.C. 20402.

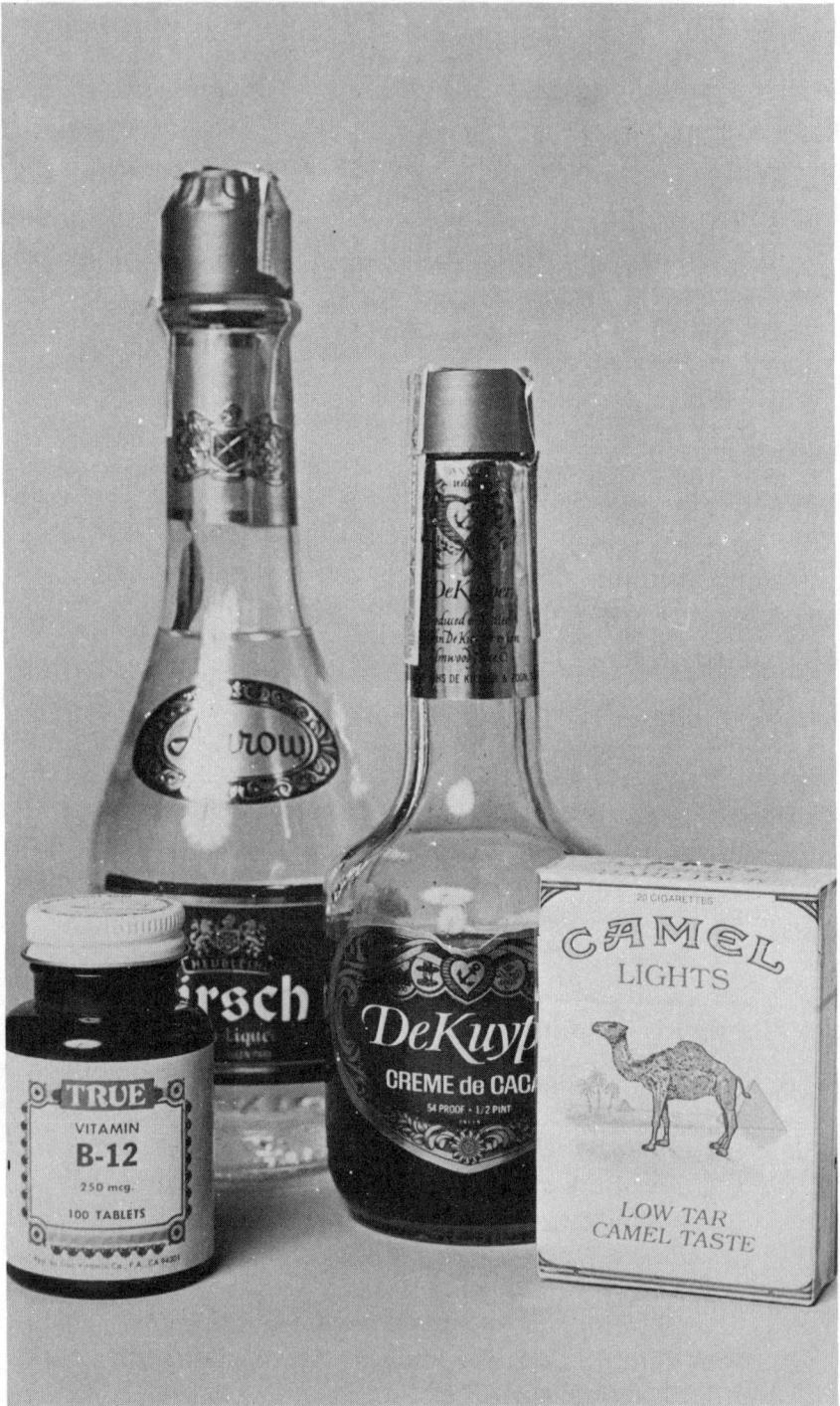

22

Drugs, Alcohol and Tobacco vs. Vitamins

DRUGS, ALCOHOL AND TOBACCO VS. VITAMINS

The human body is a large test tube into which chemicals are constantly being introduced: ascorbic acid from an orange, nitrogen in the air we breathe, monosodium glutamate in a plate of Chinese food, alcohol from a martini, and acetylsalicylic acid (aspirin) for the resulting headache. As in a test tube, the chemicals in our bodies react with one another, usually to our benefit, but occasionally to our detriment. Virtually everything that occurs in the body—from the metabolism of food into energy to the transmission of nerve impulses to the formation of flesh, blood and bones—is the direct result of chemical reactions.

As chemicals, vitamins participate in—and even catalyze—a number of these reactions. Often they're helped along with their work by minerals and other vitamins and nutrients, but occasionally they are hindered in their performance by outside chemicals. Some of these antagonists occur in the very foods we eat (i.e., oxalic acid, which binds calcium and makes it unavailable for absorption, is found in chocolate, spinach, collard greens and some other vegetables; likewise, avidin, found in uncooked egg whites, and thiaminase, found in raw clams and some other uncooked seafoods, inactivate biotin and thiamin, respectively). While, for one reason or another, such substances that occur in food have a rather insignificant effect on our vitamin supply, there are some externally imposed chemicals that can have a much greater impact. These usually come to us in the "drugs" we ingest.

171

Whether prescription, over-the-counter or illicit, drugs have the potential to influence a vitamin's performance by any of a number of means, including inhibiting its absorption, promoting its oxidation, or accelerating its excretion. One of the most direct controls drugs have over vitamin availability lies in their influence upon appetite. By suppressing appetite, for example, amphetamines, often prescribed for obesity or depression, effectively restrict the intake of food and thus of vitamins. Ingestion of a large quantity of caffeine that makes you too "wired" to eat or the practice of satisfying hunger with a saccharine-laced diet drink can perform the same function. The chemicals help keep out calories, but they also slam the door in the face of vital nutrients. Other substances—examples include B-complex liquids, chloral hydrate, some chemotherapy drugs, or even an overindulgence in alcohol—can inhibit nutrient intake by inducing nausea or gastrointestinal upset. Still others, like some antibiotics, may reduce taste sensitivity and the desire to eat.

But just because vitamins make it through the front door (i.e., actually enter the body), there is no guarantee that they'll stay long enough to accomplish their mission. Regular users of laxatives may be flushing away large quantities of unused vitamins that weren't allowed to remain in the intestines long enough to be absorbed. Along the same lines, water-soluble vitamins are speeded out of the body by the regular use of diuretic drugs, diuretic-type substances like caffeine, alcohol and nicotine, as well as by the consumption of large quantities of any kind of liquid.

Heavy consumption of alcohol is perhaps the greatest enemy of vitamins. Those who drink the equivalent of four cocktails (1½-oz. jiggers of 80-proof alcohol) per day will probably require supplementation of the water-soluble vitamins, particularly thiamin, niacin, B6 and folacin. Not only does alcohol's diuretic action speed elimination, but, as Jane Brody notes, "Alcohol damages the liver and interferes with its ability to store needed vitamins, especially folacin, and to convert the vitamins to their active chemical forms. Alcohol consumption also leads to poor absorption of vitamins from foods, and it increases the requirement for vitamins by using some to metabolize the alcohol and to repair the tissue damage it causes." Thus, even if heavy drinkers eat a well-balanced diet—which they very rarely do—they are nonetheless destroying the impact of many of the vitamins they consume.

As you might have guessed, cigarette smoking has the same

negative impact as does alcohol consumption. A Canadian study of heavy smokers (those who puff a pack-and-a-half of smokes a day) revealed they have up to 40 percent less vitamin C in their blood than non-smokers. It has been theorized that additional C is required to repair cells damaged by smoke's toxic substances. Smoking also lowers vitamin E levels.

Antibiotics such as penicillin, neomycin and tetracycline may kill more than the bug you're carrying. They can also destroy the intestinal bacteria responsible for the synthesis of vitamin K and some of the B vitamins. Absorption of the oil-soluble vitamins is affected both by mineral oil and by such drugs as cholestyramine (used to lower blood cholesterol) that bind bile salts. Anticonvulsant drugs may counteract vitamin D by increasing the activity of certain metabolic enzymes that go to work on the body's store. There are a number of vitamins that are susceptible to antacids.

Minerals, too, have their antagonists, and antacids are one of the biggest culprits. As Dr. Patricia A. Kreutler notes, those "containing aluminum inhibit absorption of phosphorus, ultimately increasing the excretion of both phosphorus and calcium; prolonged use may lead to significant demineralization of bone. The antacid property itself causes conversion of iron to insoluble and unabsorbable forms." Other undesirable combinations include phosphorus with anticonvulsants, magnesium with diuretics or alcohol, potassium with diuretics, and iron with tea.

The list of vitamins and minerals whose potency is affected by various drugs is a long one and the reasons for the adverse reactions numerous. A drug may interfere with a vitamin in a variety of ways, including damaging cells of the intestinal mucosa, interfering with transport mechanisms or causing excessive release or decreased synthesis of enzymes. We don't yet know all of the combinations of vitamin/drug interaction, nor have we begun to scratch the surface when it comes to the combinations of prescription drugs some people are required to take or the over-the-counter regimens they often prescribe for themselves.

Of course, vitamin/drug interaction is a two-sided coin. The administration of drugs is vital for serious health problems and in such cases a vitamin deficiency will have to be made up with supplementation or a change in diet. Usually the problem only presents itself when prolonged use or large doses of a drug are prescribed. Those for whom prescription drugs are an important fact of life must remember also that there are certain nutrients that can interfere with the medication they're taking. For example, a prescribed anticoagulant might be hindered by vitamin K supplementation or tetracycline lose its effectiveness in the presence of food supplements containing iron, calcium and other minerals.

For those interested in preserving vitamin and/or drug integrity, there are a couple of guidelines: 1) When prescribed a drug by your physician, question its necessity. Do you need an antibiotic to knock out that bug...or will it die a natural death in a day or two, leaving your intestinal flora intact? 2) Despite television commercials that tout tablets, time capsules and bubbly elixirs to cure everything from the morning after to a shattered romance, think twice about consuming a steady diet of the self-remedies that line the aisles of supermarkets and drug stores. 3) When your doctor prescribes a necessary drug, ask him whether it will create any special vitamin requirements or if vitamin supplements will interfere with the action of the drug. 4) Read the label on your prescription. If it contains special instructions—to take the medication with meals or to avoid taking it with dairy products, for instance—follow them.

DRUGS THAT INTERFERE WITH VITAMINS

Vitamin A — Mineral oil, cholestyramine (high blood cholesterol)* and other drugs that bind bile salts.

B1 (Thiamin) — Bicarbonate of soda, antacids, diuretics containing mercury compounds, alcohol, antibiotics;** tea.

B2 (Riboflavin) — Bicarbonate of soda, tetracycline (antibiotic), diuretics containing mercury compounds, probenecid (gout), some oral contraceptives, sulfa drugs, boric acid.

B3 (Niacin) — Alcohol, antibiotics, INH (tuberculosis), diuretics containing mercury compounds.

Biotin — Antibiotics, diuretics containing mercury compounds.

Pantothenic Acid — Bicarbonate of soda, antibiotics, diuretics containing mercury compounds.

B6 (Pyridoxine) — Oral contraceptives, INH, etc. (tuberculosis), chloramphenicol (antibiotic), hydrazide (high blood pressure) and some other diuretics, hydralazine (hypertension), penicillamine (severe arthritis).

Folacin — Aminosalicylic acid (tuberculosis), cycloserine (tuberculosis), anticonvulsants, trimethoprim (malaria), pyrimethamine (malaria), methotrexate (cancer chemotherapy), oral contraceptives, alcohol, diuretics containing mercury compounds.

B12 (Cobalamin) — Metformin (diabetes), phenformin (diabetes), bicarbonate of soda, diuretics containing mercury compounds, colchicine (gout), neomycin (antibiotic).

Vitamin C (Ascorbic acid) — Antacids, adrenal steroids, aspirin, sulfa drugs, tetracycline, tobacco, oral contraceptives,** bicarbonate of soda, diuretics containing mercury compounds, copper, iron.

Vitamin D — Mineral oil, cholestyramine, cortisone, barbiturates, anticonvulsants.

Vitamin E — Mineral oil, cholestyramine, tobacco, copper, iron.

Vitamin K — Antibiotics, anticoagulants, anticonvulsants, mineral oil, cholestyramine, aspirin.

( )* Used in the treatment of.

**Unclear.

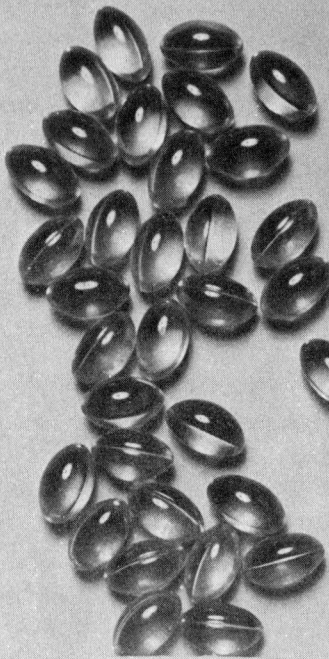

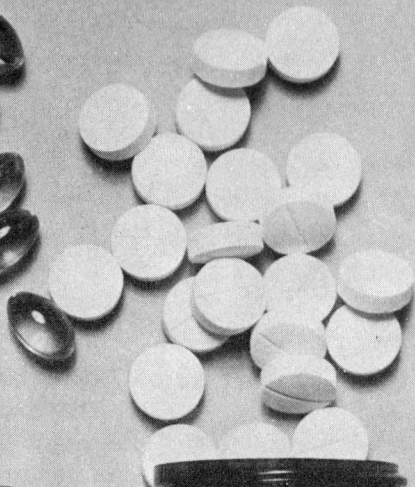

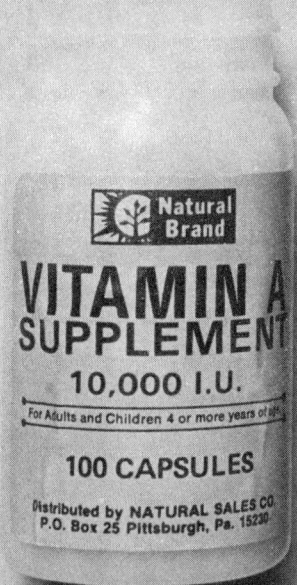

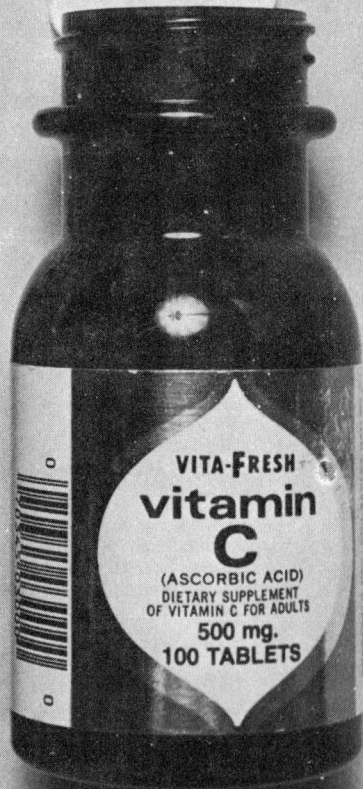

23

Picking a Pill

Once you've read the facts on the various vitamins and weighed the benefits and risks, you must decide whether you really need or want more vitamins in pill form. If the answer is yes, or if your doctor has recommended one or more vitamins, there are some things to remember about purchasing supplements.

POTENCY: The first consideration when choosing a vitamin supplement is potency. Just how much of a vitamin or vitamins do you want? Most of the once-daily multivitamins, regardless of brand, contain 100 percent or less of all of the vitamins (except K, and often with the exception of biotin). For those convinced they need the insurance of extra vitamins—a conviction the vitamin industry spends millions of advertising dollars to help you develop—a supplement of this type is more than adequate. Individuals with specific disorders might derive greater benefit from large doses of single supplements, but it is advised these be taken under the recommendation of a physician. Individual supplements (i.e., bottles of C, E, etc.) and many of the multiple vitamin combinations sold in health food stores contain much larger doses of vitamins. If you're a normal, healthy individual consuming an average diet, you don't need any of these, unless you are trying to reap benefits that are not yet known to exist. If you are convinced that extra vitamins are for you, be very careful of dosage. This is particularly important with the vitamins that have the greatest toxicity potential. Just because something is on the market, doesn't mean it's safe (remember that 25,000 IU vitamin A supplement) and even if there were limitations on the potency of vitamin tablets, no one could control the number of tablets you take.

Be aware particularly of potency of individual vitamins in health food store multivitamins. Like the manufacturer who decided according to his own evidence that we need seven times the RDA for vitamin A, manufacturers often have their own rhyme-and-reasonless formulas for determining the amounts of vitamins that go into multis. Sometimes these formulations are based on nothing more scientific than the relative cost of individual vitamins; i.e., you get more of the cheap ones, less of the expensive ones. While such formulas may contain some vitamins in amounts closely approximating the RDA, they may have much greater quantities of others. Some may contain many times the RDA for all of the vitamins. As we know, that's probably fine for some of the vitamins, but could cause trouble with others. Check the potency of every vitamin in such a formula to see if they exceed the maximum amounts you're willing to take a chance on.

Another thing to remember is that vitamins may actually have more than their stated potency. According to the authors of *The Vitamin Book,* many manufacturers follow the practice of "including in supplements more than the labeled amount of some vitamins to ensure the vitamins' stated potency throughout its shelf life. For example, the overage may be as high as 40 percent for vitamin A; that is, a supplement with a labeled dose of 25,000 IU may provide as much as 35,000 IU."

Thus, you cannot just walk into a store and pull a supplement off the shelf and expect it to be the same as all the rest in terms of potency. Most vitamins come in different strengths (i.e., 50,100, 250, 500 and 1000 mg tablets of C), and multiple vitamins often vary widely in their concentrations of individual vitamins. Read the label to assure you're not getting more than you bargained for....or that you're getting the full strength your doctor prescribed. And make sure you don't confuse milligrams (mg) with micrograms (mcg).

FORM: Vitamins come in a host of configurations, including tablets, capsules, liquids and powders. Powders are probably the least common and most potent form, since they are often straight vitamin without the binders, fillers, etc., needed to hold tablets together. Tablets are merely glued-together versions of powders that are more convenient for most people to take. Likewise, gelatin capsules contain either powdered vitamin or oil-suspended A, D or E. In the latter case, the capsule helps you avoid the unpleasant taste and texture of the vegetable or fish oil in which the vitamin is dissolved. Liquid supplements are most often used for infants, children and those who have trouble swallowing pills. Vitamin C and children's vitamin supplements also commonly appear in chewable "candy" form. While, perhaps, painless and palatable, remember that these contain sugar and lots of fillers. The advice in Earl Mindell's dubiously titled *Vitamin Bible* aside, don't be fooled into paying more for so-called "better brands" of these vitamins that use fructose, honey and other sweeteners in place of "sugar." Sugar is sugar regardless of its source and all types (honey, sucrose, etc.) have the same number of empty calories, promote tooth decay and function the same way in the body. Remember, also, that supplements in this form really *are not* candy....and make sure you don't promote them to your children that way. Children have suffered vitamin and iron poisoning as a result of polishing off a bottle of these tasty little goodies shaped like cute animals and cartoon characters. It is important to keep all vitamin supplements tightly capped and out of the reach of children. There are thousands of cases of vitamin poisoning reported each year involving the youthful set. Another more insidious type of harm children's supplements can do is to give youngsters the false impression that there is a magic health pill. Far too many of us grow up believing in panaceas that will make up for our poor eating habits and lack of knowledge about nutrition. If parents wanted to do their children a real service, they would forget about candy-coated supplements and provide their children with a wide variety of fresh, whole foods. Good eating habits formed early on will serve your child well throughout his life.

TIME RELEASE: If large quantities of water-soluble vitamins B and C are ingested at once, most of them will be flushed out of the body within a very short time. Time-release capsules are designed to give you a constant supply of the vitamin at an even rate throughout the day....without the inconvenience of taking a pill more than once.

Time release capsules are formulated in three basic ways. One procedure calls for mixing particles of the vitamin in carnuba wax (well, it works for your car doesn't it?), which is then allowed to harden. Since the wax breaks down slowly in the body, the tablet slowly dissolves, releasing the vitamin into the body.

Another method produces a layered tablet in which successive layers of the vitamin are covered with shellac (food glaze) or zein corn protein. As each layer of coating is dissolved, the layer of vitamin below is exposed.

The third and most common time-release form is the Contac-like beadlet-filled capsule. According to one manufacturer, the "Beadlets can be simply formed by combining the nutrient with a filler such as dicalcium phosphate and shellac. The paste formed by these combined ingredients is then forced through an extruder in order to produce long noodles. The noodles are subsequently tumbled in a stainless steel drum where they break apart. The tumbling action also forms the noodle fragments into rounded beadlets. The beadlets are then dried and may be encapsulated in two-piece hard-shell capsules or combined with more nutrient and excipients and pressed into a conventional tablet shape."

The general manager of one large vitamin company says his firm makes no claims for the benefits of time-release tablets because there have been no studies to show if they are helpful. They are made, he says, because of customer demand.

The third trial conducted by Terence Anderson and his colleagues, to test the effectiveness of vitamin C against the common cold, shed some light on the time-release issue: "Half of the vitamin subjects," says Anderson, "received a sustained-release form of the vitamin that should be more efficiently retained (and therefore possibly equivalent to higher dose) than an ordinary tablet, since it avoids the rapid absorption and excretion seen with the conventional tablet form of dose. However, there was no striking difference in the results observed with the two types of vitamin dosage...."

Before you pay at least twice as much for time-release tablets or capsules, consider whether you might not rather take smaller amounts of vitamin C at various intervals throughout the day. Better yet, consider whether time-release might not be just another way to more effectively use what you don't really need.

STORAGE: Even under ideal storage conditions, vitamins lose some or all of their potency with age. You can slow down the process—certainly for the time it takes to get through a bottle of supplements—by storing your vitamins tightly capped in an opaque bottle. Keep in a cool, dry, dark place.

UNNECESSARY INGREDIENTS: To save money and still get what you need, avoid the extraneous ingredients that are the order of the day in many health food store supplements, as well as the myriad products aimed at the athlete. A vitamin/mineral supplement must contain vitamins and minerals—a total of about twelve to seventeen of them—and that's it. Some manufacturers—those who produce the so-called "natural" brands are the worst offender—like to convince you that you need lots of little extras to make you work better. As Sidney Margolius reports in *Health Foods: Facts and Fakes*, supplements sometimes contain as many as seventy-five such ingredients. You can buy tablets with anything you want—or don't want—from kelp to pectin, but most of these ingredients are substances for which your body has no need. In *Vitamins And You*, Robert J. Benowicz has an interesting perspective on the practice of packing pills with extra goodies:

> "The fundamental belief that 'more must be better' is often exploited by vitamin shysters who may pack their products with extraneous ingredients and charge an exorbitant price for the excess baggage. The inclusion of such exotica as amino acids (e.g., lysine, betaine, glutamic acid, etc.), enzymes, RNA, chlorophyll, essential fatty acids, and the like in a supplement is a sure sign of hucksterism. Look for products containing only the vitamins and minerals you need."

SPECIAL FORMULATIONS: Many vitamin companies manufacture products geared to those with allergies or diet restrictions. Ask a clerk to show you which lines are made without corn, dairy, wheat or animal products if you are excluding any of these from your diet.

LABELING: If there is something you don't want in a vitamin—i.e., sugar, colorings, flavorings, preservatives—don't assume it isn't there unless the label flatly states it isn't. These substances are particularly prevalent in chewable vitamins.

PRICE: A price difference between two brands of vitamins with identical ingredients may mean that the company charging more practices stricter quality control. Usually it means that the company's marketing staff decided they could get away with a higher price or reflects a bigger advertising budget, fancy packaging or some other gimmick. Many brands sold door-to-door are exorbitantly priced not because of their superiority, but because they are marketed through a pyramid distributorship system that makes it necessary for dozens of people to get a cut from each sale. In most cases, you have no way of knowing why one supplement costs more than another. As Benowicz says, "Higher prices are typical of products from the major pharmaceutical houses. Choose such supplements if you feel more comfortable with a well-known brand name behind you, but remember that unfamiliar or generically labeled products probably provide you with equivalent quality and greater value for your dollar." Actually, many different vitamin brands contain the very same substance, purchased from the same major vitamin manufacturer; for example, as much as 70 percent of the bulk vitamins sold in the U.S. and the free world come from Hoffman-LaRoche, those fun people who brought you Valium. Generally, the ingredients on the label being equal, you might as well go with the cheaper brand. It isn't always easy to determine which one that is, however. Those random formulations we talked about earlier make it hard to compare prices of multivitamin supplements. Also, there are some brands that make it look as though you are getting many more pills for the price, but if you read the label you will learn that three tablets a day are required to do the job of one tablet of a slightly more expensive brand.

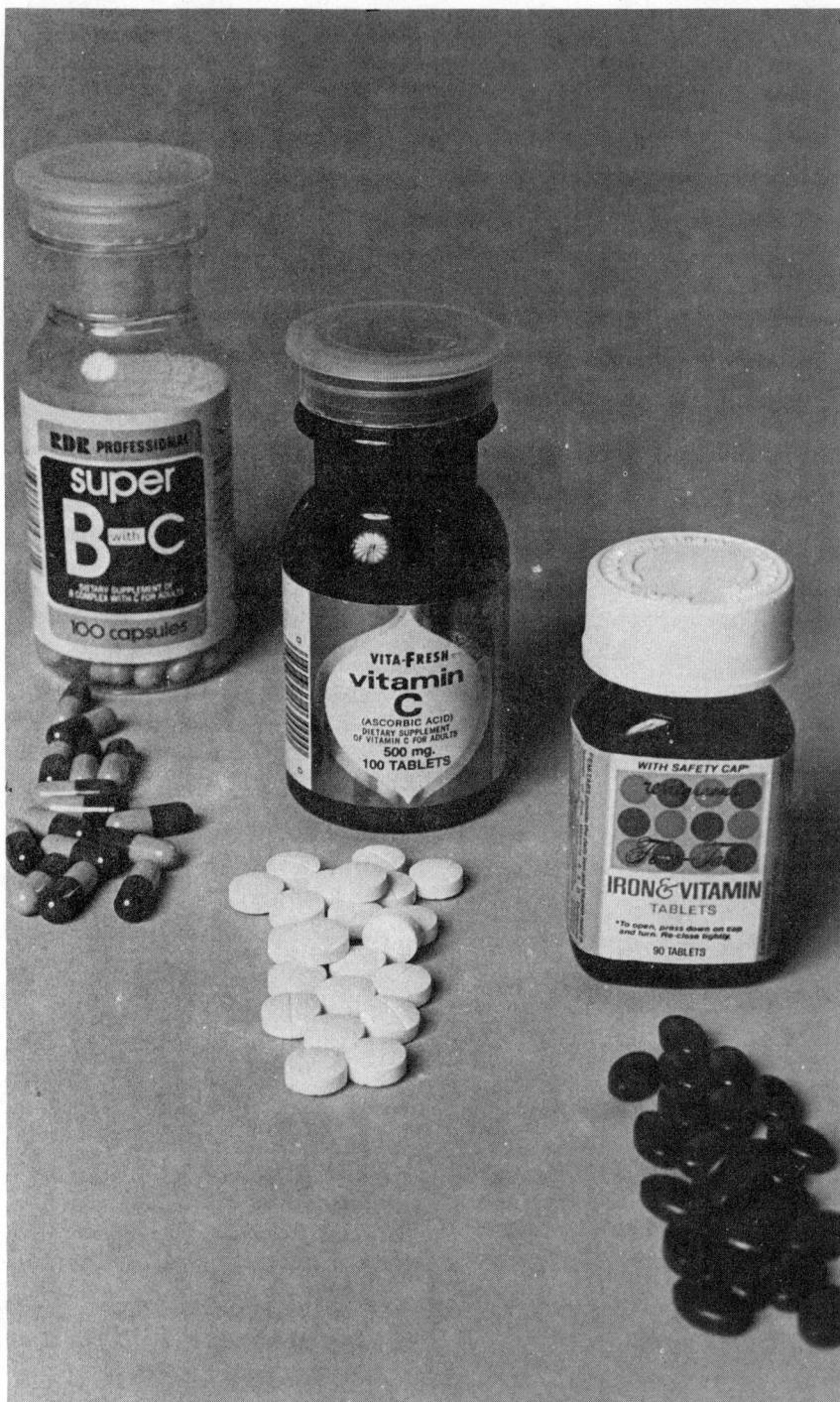

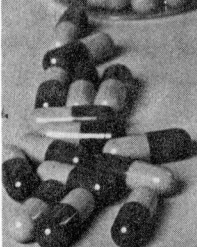

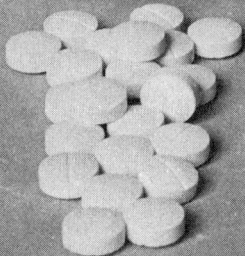

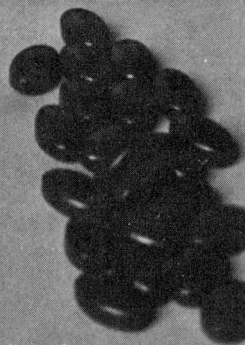

24

Natural Vitamins vs. Synthetic

One of the biggest decisions facing the vitamin buyer is whether to purchase a "natural" brand or a "synthetic" one at less than half the price. If you want to know the reasons why natural vitamins are so far superior to synthetic vitamins, it is only necessary to ask a clerk in a health food store. Unfortunately, very little that you hear will be true. It isn't so much a matter of dishonesty as one of misinformation. There are dozens of arguments used by proponents of "natural" vitamins, many of which sound very logical and convincing. It's a good idea to go into some of them, but first it is important to know what we mean by the terms "natural," "synthetic" and "organic."

"Natural" generally refers to vitamins extracted from natural sources; i.e., vitamin C taken from an orange is natural. "Synthetic" refers to vitamins that are synthesized or compounded in the laboratory. "Organic," which is commonly used by makers of food and vitamins alike, conjures up visions of a fresh, wholesome product that comes, unsullied, straight from nature. In truth, the term "organic" simply refers to any chemical compound containing carbon. Thus, as biochemist Robert J. Benowicz points out, "Coal tar, plastics, and petroleum products all qualify but hardly fulfill the expectations aroused." Continues Benowicz, "When applied to a vitamin supplement, the term 'organic' simply means that a portion of the product has been extracted from plant or animal tissue. It is rare for a label to indicate what proportion of a vitamin comes from such tissue or what extraction processes were employed in retrieval." According to Marilyn Stephenson, an FDA nutritionist, her agency has taken no position on the use of such terms as "organic," "natural" and "health" in labeling because

185

they are so loosely and interchangeably used. She goes on to say that the Federal Trade Commission would like to prohibit use of the words "organic" and "natural" in advertising because of concern about the ability of consumers to understand the terms in the conflicting and confusing ways they are used. Ask the average person who is paying extra for "natural" or "organic" products exactly what he is getting and chances are he won't be able to tell you. That's just the way the manufacturers like it.

Are natural vitamins different from or superior to synthetic ones? In *The Health Robbers,* Dr. Victor Herbert pulls no punches when he says, "This claim is a flat lie and anyone who makes it should be immediately classified by you as a quack. Each vitamin is a chain of atoms strung together as a molecule. Molecules made in the "factories" of nature are identical to those made in the factories of chemical companies."

Dr. Carol Grimes, professor of chemistry and nutrition at Goldenwest College, agrees that the question is one of molecular identity: "Let's say I make ascorbic acid in the lab (which, incidentally, one makes from glucose, which one can get from natural sources so when do you draw the line about calling something natural versus synthetic?), purify it and put it in a test tube labeled just 'ascorbic acid' and hand it to another chemist. Then I isolate some from oranges, for example, purify it and hand it to the same chemist. If I ask him to tell me which one came from which source, it turns out he can't. There is no physical or chemical test that one can apply that will tell the molecules apart. We cannot tell them apart in that way." Neither, it turns out, can our bodies. In fact, if the synthetic substance were chemically different from the natural one, it would no longer be ascorbic acid and could not, by law, be sold as such.

Because vitamins from natural sources have no nutritional superiority over synthetic vitamins, the FDA prohibits such claims in labeling. Ironically, however, that agency has not been able to crack down on use of the terms "organic" and "natural" on products that may actually contain synthetic substances. The reason is probably one of the most convincing arguments for the fact that synthetic and natural vitamins are chemically identical: According to Adolph Kamil, pharmacist of the Consumers Co-Operative of Berkeley and assistant clinical professor of pharmacology at the University of California Medical Center, "Apparently, these words can be used freely because there are no legal definitions of 'natural' or 'organic.' In fact, since the vitamins themselves are identical, no one can tell them apart—either in a test tube cr in an animal. A legal distinction could hardly be enforced when no way can be devised to test the difference."

If the two types of vitamins are not different, why do health food advocates claim that one is better than the other? For those in the supplements business, the reason is obvious: most of us believe in the natural vitamin myth and not only prefer the products labeled this way, but are willing to pay two, three or many times more for them. Aside from the current widespread belief that anything "natural" is inherently superior to anything manmade (think for a moment of the stigma attached to anything polyester), one argument most of us buy is that synthetic vitamins may be contaminated by toxic substances left over from the manufacturing process. According to Dr. Grimes, "Our methods of detection for this sort of thing are very, very precise and pharmaceutical-grade chemicals are very, very pure." Drs. Joseph V. Levy and Paul Bach-y-Rita, authors of *Vitamins: Their Use and Abuse*, concur: "The purity and identity of (the chemist's) efforts can be checked and confirmed by precise methods which can detect contamination, impurities or instability. Exact qualities that must be met to satisfy the label 'Vitamin C,' or ascorbic acid, for use in humans, are defined by the United States Pharmacopoeia Commission."

If we are worried about "unnatural" substances in our vitamin supplements, we must worry about natural vitamins, as well. As Benowicz points out, "The extraction process itself may require use of the very same harsh solvents, high heat and pressure that, by implication, are so assiduously avoided in compounding a product." Kamil, who, spurred by growing sales of natural vitamins at the Berkeley Co-Op, visited Southern California manufacturers of these substances in an effort to find out more about them, learned this about two manufacturers' vitamin E products: "Vitamin E products are indeed derived from natural sources—mainly vegetable oils such as wheat germ, soy bean and corn. These are sold as cheaply as the synthetic variety, but, in order to concentrate the vitamin in a capsule small enough to swallow, various chemical solvents must be used for extraction and separation. The vegetable material is grown with the use of the usual insecticides and chemical fertilizers. Even the gelatin capsule must contain a preservative so that it won't turn rancid."

To add further to the "unnaturalness" of "natural" products, fillers, binders and other substances don't have to be listed on labels and most often aren't. Thus, you often have no idea what is used to dry, lubricate, color, flavor, disintegrate, deodorize, bind or fill your natural vitamins. Most often they are the same ingredients found in synthetic brands. On top of that, there are many toxicants (i.e., lead, arsenic, cyanide, cadmium, etc.) that occur naturally in foods. While these may occur in harmless quantities in food, they can reach much higher levels in concentrates made from that food.

Another thing that is claimed specifically for some things like ascorbic acid is that perhaps there is some accompanying substance in the natural preparation of the vitamin which makes it better absorbed and utilized. For example, in his *Vitamin Bible*, Earl Mindell maintains that "Synthetic vitamin C is just that, ascorbic acid and nothing more. Natural vitamin C from rose hips contains bioflavonoids, the entire C complex, which make the C much more effective." According to Dr. Grimes, one of the bioflavonoids, rutin, has been shown to improve the absorption and utilization of ascorbic acid in guinea pigs. Experiments in human beings, however, have not shown that to be true. There are, especially where vitamins are concerned, very real differences between species.

Others have argued that if there are as yet unknown vitamins or other necessary substances that remain intact in vitamins extracted from natural sources, they must be required by the body in very miniscule amounts, because, as *The Vitamin Book* suggests, "no evidence of deficiency diseases which respond to specific foods or natural vitamin supplements have been found." Dr. Grimes advises that the possible existence of these "unknown substances" or substances whose *function* is unknown is just one more good reason to obtain our vitamins from the foods we eat. "Wouldn't it be better to eat a broad variety of foods and try to make sure you get any unknown substance there?" Thus, if you want rutin with your vitamin C, why buy an exorbitantly priced natural supplement when you can get it—and over 65 mg of vitamin C—by eating an orange?

Some proponents of natural vitamins have used rather misleading illustrations to demonstrate the superiority of this type of vitamin. Often they back up their claims with results that pit synthetic vitamins against whole natural foods. As Margolius points out, "This is somewhat different from comparing synthetic vitamins with vitamins isolated from the foods. The actual foods, of course, have additional vitamins and nutrients, and presumably a more natural balance of them....In one such comparison, *Prevention* stated that minks 'fed all known B vitamins in synthetic form....would eventually die (but) fed yeast, however, they stay healthy and beautifully furred on its natural B complex.' The magazine omitted the fact that the yeast is also very rich in protein; iron, calcium, and other minerals; and also provides other vitamins." Read the so-called health magazines closely and you will find them rife with such faulty reasoning and inaccurate extrapolations from animal studies. Such publications do have their uses: they keep health food store shelves stocked with expensive "natural" vitamins from manufacturers who take out ads in health food magazines.

In the continuing struggle to prove the superiority of natural vitamins, some have argued that chromatograms of synthetic vitamin C show it to be uniform and symmetrical in appearance, while natural C has irregular surfaces and edges. Say Levy and Bach-y-Rita, "This difference is always interpreted in favor of the 'natural' vitamin, i.e., it 'looks alive,' etc. What is never mentioned is the fact that such irregularities suggest chemical impurity or presence of other substances, which reflect a pattern more complex than the pure synthetic material." Benowicz adds that "Evidence indicates that extraction of organic or natural forms is often incomplete and does not always yield the pure vitamin. That the residue of such processes contains an unknown, but vital, nutritional factor cannot be confirmed. That such impurity may interfere with proper intestinal absorption of the vitamin *can* be substantiated."

If you are convinced that natural vitamins are somehow better for you, make sure you're getting what you think you're paying for. For some vitamins (E, for example), extraction from natural sources is more efficient and less expensive than starting from scratch, so virtually all of that vitamin—cheap or expensive—is "natural."

For other vitamins, extraction from nature is much more costly....perhaps the reason we find it much more desirable. Labels are not required to state the source of the vitamins contained inside, and very few do. Ascorbic acid can—and should be—called ascorbic acid no matter where it comes from....and most often it comes from the laboratory.

We are all convinced of the superior benefits of vitamin C extracted from rose hips. But how many of us have ever wondered why? Apparently they were first used as a source of the vitamin during World War II in Great Britain and Canada, where oranges don't grow, but roses thrive. According to Marion McGill and Orrea Pye in *The No-Nonsense Guide to Food & Nutrition*, "During the War, rose hips were promoted as a source of vitamin C to avoid the necessity of importing citrus fruits. They are not particularly exciting to eat and are no match for a glass of fresh orange juice or half a papaya. Dried, as sold in health food stores, they are a dubious source of vitamin C." Perhaps it's the exotic-sounding name that makes many of us feel that the seed pods of roses, once used only out of necessity, are the best source of vitamin C. But what we don't realize is that rose hips have only about 2 percent vitamin C and that in order to get a few hundred milligrams of vitamin C from rose hips we would have to swallow a pill larger than a golf ball. Most natural vitamins get around remaining natural by adding rose hips to synthetic ascorbic acid and calling the product Rose Hips Vitamin C or Vitamin C with Rose Hips. But even if the product is a 50/50 mixture—100 milligrams of ascorbic acid and 100 milligrams of rose hips, you're only getting 102 milligrams of vitamin C....and only 2 percent of that is from rose hips. Similarly, just because you spend more to buy vitamin C that includes acerola (from expensive acerola cherries—how's that for exotic?), promoted as containing "up to 80 times more vitamin C than an equal amount of orange juice," you're still only getting 100 mg of vitamin in a 100 mg tablet. And 100 mg of vitamin C from one source is the same as that from another.

In his visit to the natural vitamin companies, Kamil found it to be the case that most products (B-complexes, for example), were mostly things like yeast extracts added to synthetic B vitamins. In a recent article on vitamins as big business, *Forbes* magazine printed the following quote from a vitamin company manager: "Look, people want 'natural' and will pay a premium for it, so why not give it to them? If you made a whole vitamin C tablet from rose hips, say, either your cost to extract it would be prohibitive or the size of the pill would be too big to swallow. Marketers aren't stupid. They include a minor fraction of ascorbic acid from rose hips, give it a 'natural' sounding brand name, and put some brown flecks in so it looks like the stuff was just swept up off a dirt floor. Read the labels sometime."

While that may be the prevailing attitude of the "natural" vitamin industry, perhaps the occasional ray of light shed on the true situation will give rise to another. Take for example, this account from *FDA Consumer:* "Recently it was reported that a natural food store in California removed all vitamins, which are high profit items, from its shelves. The management had learned that most of a product labeled "Rose Hips Vitamin C from Natural Sources" was synthetic. Unable to confirm that similar practices do not occur in other natural vitamin supplements, the store stopped handling vitamins and suggested that people get them from a pharmacy where the pills aren't labeled as natural and they're cheaper."

Many of us have jumped on the natural vitamins, natural foods, natural everything bandwagon with good intentions. We're tired of over-processed empty foods that provide calories but little nutrition. Likewise, startled by reports of chemicals that can cause this or that disease, we've come to shudder at the thought of anything that comes from a test tube. Those reactions are understandable and the quest for wholesome foods is an admirable one. But somewhere in the process we have grown to mistrust the whole foods we can still buy and to worship the pills we think are made from them. At the same time we have lost sight of the fact that vitamins are chemicals no matter where they occur and as such can be exactly duplicated in the laboratory.

In fact, what has happened is that those of us who were tired of being cheated by plastic foods, have given rise to a whole new kind of hucksterism. We've become the natural generation who are suckers for anything with the words "natural," "organic" or "health" on the label. Big business, as always, has been quick to comply with our wishes, because, as marketing surveys reveal, one of those words on the label can assure that a product is a best-seller. Just like magic its addition to a package can turn whatever is inside—from beer to potato chips—into something that's good for us. Similarly, it can make one of two identical products superior and therefore more expensive.

When it comes to food, it isn't misguided to want the whole, natural stuff—the fresh fruits, vegetables, meats, dairy products, grains, etc. When it comes to vitamins, it isn't misguided to want the same thing. And if that is the case, we'll do well to remember that the ultimate in natural vitamins is not those taken—or supposedly taken—from yeast or oranges or liver, but the fresh, whole foods themselves.

COMPARATIVE PRICES OF
NATURAL AND SYNTHETIC VITAMIN E *

NAME & INGREDIENTS	POTENCY	NO. OF TABLETS	PRICE	COST PER 100 IU
HEALTH FOOD STORE NATURAL BRAND				
Naturade Mixed Tocopherols Vitamin E	200 IU	100	$6.50	$0.032

Ingred.: "Each capsule contains 200 IU of vitamin E (d-alpha-tocopherol) from a preparation containing mixed tocopherols derived from natural vegetable oils."

| **DOOR-TO-DOOR/DISTRIB-UTORSHIP NATURAL BRAND** | | | | |
| Shaklee Vita-E Tablets Plus Selenium | 100 IU** | 100 | $9.15 | $0.091 |

Ingred.: "d-alpha-tocopheryl acetate, dicalcium phosphate, sorbitol, mannitol, selenium yeast, fructose, wheat germ flour, mixed tocopherol concentrate, colored with turmeric, natural flavor."

| **NATIONALLY ADVERTISED DRUGSTORE SYNTHETIC BRAND** | | | | |
| Squibb Vitamin E Dietary Supplement (artifical walnut flavored) | 200 IU | 100 | $6.29 | $0.031 |

Ingred.: "Sugar, gelatin, dl-a-tocopheryl acetate, invert sugar, silica gel, artificial flavors, magnesium stearate, colloidal silicon dioxide, FD&C Yellow No. 5, sodium benzoate and sorbic acid as preservatives, corn starch.

| **SUPERMARKET GENERIC SYNTHETIC BRAND** | | | | |
| Safeway Vitamin E Supplement | 200 IU | 100 | $2.99 | $0.014 |

Ingred.: "dl-alphatocopherol acetate, gelatin, glycerin, natural vegetable (soybean) oil, methyl and propyl parabens as preservatives and artificial flavor."

| **SUPERMARKET GENERIC NATURAL BRAND** | | | | |
| Safeway Vitamin E Supplement*** | 200 IU | 90 | $4.79 | $0.026 |

Ingred.: "soybean oil, dl-alpha-tocopherol acetate, gelatin, glycerin, water, methylparaben and propylparaben as preservatives."

DRUGSTORE GENERIC
SYNTHETIC BRAND
Thrifty Drug
Vitamin E   200 IU   100 $3.19 $0.015

Ingred.: "Each capsule contains 200 IU of Vitamin E from dl-alpha-tocopheryl acetate."

DRUGSTORE GENERIC
NATURAL BRAND
Thrifty Drug Natural
Vitamin E Supplement   100 IU   100 $3.29 $0.032

Ingred.: "Preparation of d-alpha tocopheryl acetate N.F. containing 73.5 mg d-alpha tocopheryl acetate and blend of vegetable oils (soybean and corn oil), plus gelatin, glycerin, with methyl and propyl parabens as a preservative, and artificial flavors."

*The U.S. RDA for vitamin E is 30 IU.

**It is necessary to read this label carefully. Nowhere on the label is the per tablet potency stated. The unit of measure and % of U.S. RDA are stated on the ingredients panel as 300 IU and 1000 percent, respectively. Only here do we learn that this is the amount supplied by *three* tablets.

***The label on this product does not state that it is the company's "natural" brand; that is only implied by the label art and the higher price.

Bibliography

BOOKS

Adams, Catherine F. *Nutritive Value of American Foods* (Agriculture Handbook No. 456). Washington, D.C.: Agricultural Research Service, USDA, 1975.

Adams, Ruth. *The Complete Home Guide To All The Vitamins.* NY: Larchmont Books, 1976.

Bailey, Herbert. *Vitamin E: Your Key To A Healthy Heart.* NY: Arc Books, 1968.

Barrett, Stephen and Gilda Knight. *The Health Robbers.* Philadelphia: George F. Stickley, 1976.

Benowicz, Robert J. *Vitamins & You.* NY: Grosset & Dunlap, 1979.

Brody, Jane. *Jane Brody's Nutrition Book.* NY: W.W. Norton, 1981.

Consumer Guide. *The Vitamin Book.* NY: Simon & Schuster, 1979.

Consumer Reports. *The Medicine Show.* Mount Vernon, NY: Consumers Union, 1970.

Culbert, Michael L. *Freedom From Cancer: The Amazing Story of Laetrile.* Seal Beach, CA: Seventy-Six Press, 1976.

Dicyan, Erwin. *Vitamin E & Aging.* NY: Jove Publications, 1972.

Hausman, Patricia. *Jack Sprat's Legacy: The Science and Politics of Fat & Cholesterol.* NY: Richard Marek Publishers, 1981.

Kreutler, Patricia A. *Nutrition In Perspective.* Englewood Cliffs, NJ: Prentice-Hall, 1980.

Labuza, Theodore P., ed. *The Nutrition Crisis.* St. Paul: West Publishing Co., 1975. (Collected reprints on vitamins, etc.)

Labuza, Theodore P. and A. Elizabeth Sloan, eds. *Contemporary Nutrition Controversies.* St. Paul: West Publishing Co., 1979. (Collected reprints on vitamins, etc.).

Levy, Joseph V. and Paul Bach-y-Rita. *Vitamins: Their Use And Abuse.* NY: Liveright, 1976.

Mindell, Earl. *Vitamin Bible.* NY: Rawson, Wade Publishers, 1980.

Margolius, Sidney. *Health Foods: Facts and Fakes.* NY: Walker & Co., 1973.

McGill, Marion and Orrea Pye. *The No-Nonsense Guide To Food And Nutrition.* NY: Butterick Publishing, 1978.

National Research Council, Food and Nutrition Board. *Recommended Dietary Allowances,* 9th ed. Washington, D.C.: National Academy of Sciences, 1980.

Prevention Magazine. *The Complete Book of Vitamins.* Emmaus, PA: Rodale Press, 1977.

Risenberg, Harold. *The Doctor's Book of Vitamin Therapy.* NY: G.P. Putnam's Sons, 1974.

Watt, Bernice K. and Annabel L. Merrill. *Composition of Foods* (Agriculture Handbook No. 8). Washington, D.C.: Consumer and Food Economics Research Division, Agricultural Research Service, USDA, 1963.

Wentzler, Rich. *The Vitamin Book.* Garden City, NY: Doubleday & Co., 1979.

Williams, Roger J. *Nutrition Against Disease.* NY: Bantam Books, 1973.

Williams, Sue Rodwell. *Nutrition And Diet Therapy.* 3rd ed. St. Louis: C.V. Mosby Co., 1977.

Zimmerman, Caroline A. *Laetrile: Hope–Or Hoax?* NY: Zebra Books, 1977.

ARTICLES

Anon. "Sense and Nonsense About Vitamins." *Changing Times,* March 1980, p. 53.

Anon. "Shaklee: Curbing Profits To Gain New Vigor In the Vitamin Market." *Business Week,* 9 June 1980, p. 108.

Anon. "Vitamins: Gear Their Intake To Your Special Needs." *Science Digest,* July 1979, p. 82.

Benowicz, Robert J. "Age of Vitamins." *Family Health,* Sept. 1980, p. 28.

Benowicz, Robert J. "In Buying Supplements Be Sure of Your A-B6-and-Cs." *Science Digest,* Nov. 1979, p. 73.

Bieri, J.G. "Vitamin E." Reprinted from *Nutrition Reviews,* June 1975, p. 161.

Bruck, C. "Vitamins." *New Times,* 24 July 1978, p. 54.

Creagan, E.T., et. al. "Failure of High Dose Vitamin C (Ascorbic Acid) Therapy To Benefit Patients With Advanced Cancer." Rptd. from *New England Journal of Medicine,* 27 Sept. 1979, p. 687.

Darby, William J., Kristen W. McNutt and E. Neige Todhunter. "Niacin." Rptd. from *Nutrition Reviews,* Oct. 1975, p. 289.

DeLuca, H.F. "The Vitamin D System In the Regulation of Calcium and Phosphorus Metabolism." Rptd. from *Nutrition Reviews,* June 1979, p. 161.

DeMoss, Virginia. "Good, The Bad And The Edible." *Runner's World,* June 1980, p. 42.

Deutsch, Ronald M. "Food Fads: Fantasy and Fact." In "Food & Fitness." Chicago: Blue Cross Assoc., 1973.

Emmett, A. "Are You Overdosing On Vitamins?" *Ms.,* August 1978, p. 13.

Halsted, Charles H. "The Small Intestine In Vitamin B12 and Folate Deficiency." Rptd. from *Nutrition Reviews,* Feb. 1975, p. 33.

Senator Hatch. "Voluntary Vitamins Act of 1981." *Congressional Record–Senate,* 11 June 1981.

Haussler, Mark R. "Vitamin D: Mode of Action and Biomedical Applications." Rptd. from *Nutrition Reviews,* Sept. 1974, p. 257.

Horwitt, M.K. "Therapeutic Uses of Vitamin E In Medicine." Rptd. from *Nutrition Reviews,* March 1980, p. 105.

Kaercher, Dan. "Are You Getting Enough Vitamins?" *Better Homes & Gardens,* June 1981, p. 90.

Kamil, Adolph. "How Natural Are Those 'Natural' Vitamins?" Rptd. from *Nutrition Reviews*, July 1974, p. 34.

Lehmann, Phyllis. "Vitamania." *Vogue*, Nov. 1978, p. 196.

Lehmann, Phyllis. "Vitamin Facts and Fads." *Sciquest*, May/June 1980, p. 7.

M.L.S. "When Vitamins Can Kill." *Good Housekeeping*, June 1981, p. 218.

Mayer, Jean. "Megavitamin Madness: How Much Is Too Much?" *Family Health*, Feb. 1980, p. 48.

McCormick, Donald B. "Biotin." Rptd. from *Nutrition Reviews*, April 1975, p. 97.

Mickelsen, Olaf. "Vitamin E—Fact or Fiction?" *Nutrition Viewpoint* (Bulletin 740), Michigan State University, 1973.

Morgenstern, D. "Truth About Natural Vitamins." *McCalls*, August 1979, p. 54.

Sencker, H. "Body Building At Hoffman-LaRoche." *Forbes*, 5 Feb. 1979, p. 92.

Stein, Jane. "Vitamins: How Much Is Too Much?" *McCalls*, Nov. 1979, p. 129.

Tannenhaus, N. "Vitamins: Can They Cure Disease, Boost Energy and Jazz Up Your Sex Life?" *Glamour*, May 1979, p. 270.

PAMPHLETS AND PAPERS

American Cancer Society. "Laetrile," 1971.

American Cancer Society. "Laetrile: Background Information," 1977.

American Cancer Society. "Unproven Methods of Cancer Management," 1979.

American Medical Association. "Your Age and Your Diet," 1979.

American Psychiatric Association. "Megavitamin and Orthomolecular Therapy in Psychiatry," 1974.

Brown, Helene. "Cancer Quakery: What You Can Do About It." Rptd. from *Nursing 75* by American Cancer Society, 1975.

Committee on Nutritional Misinformation. "Selenium And Human Health." National Academy of Sciences, 1976.

Committee on Nutritional Misinformation. "Soil Fertility and the Nutritive Value of Crops." National Academy of Sciences, Sept. 1976.

Consumer and Food Economics Institute. "Nutritive Value of Foods" (Home and Garden Bulletin No. 72). USDA, 1964.

DeVita, Vincent T. "Cancer Treatment." U.S. Dept. of Health and Human Services/Public Health Service/National Institutes of Health.

FAO Nutritional Studies/WHO Monograph Series. "Handbook on Human Nutritional Requirements." Food and Agriculture Organization of the U.N., 1974.

Hayes, K.C. and D. Mark Hegsted. "Toxicity of the Vitamins."

Hausman, Patricia. "Vitamin Therapy in Degenerative Disease," 9 Dec. 1977.

Katz, Marcella. "Vitamins, Food and Your Health" (Public Affairs Pamphlet No. 465). NY: Public Affairs Committee, 1971.

Kovaly, Kenneth A. "The Vitamin Story," Stamford, CT: Good Reading Rack Service, 1971.

Levy, Robert I. "Heart Attacks." U.S. Dept. of Health, Education & Welfare, 1980.

Mindell, Earl. "Vitamins Are Good For You," 1978.

National Cancer Institute. "Statement on Diet, Nutrition and Cancer, Oct. 1979.

National Cancer Institute. "What You Need To Know About Cancer," (DHEW Publication No. (NIH) 79-1566).

National Dairy Council. "Vitamin Facts." 1981.

Ross Laboratories. "Cancer: Dietary Modification In Disease," Oct. 1978.

Shimkin, Michael B. "Science and Cancer" (NIH Pub. 80-568). National Cancer Institute/U.S. Dept. of Health and Human Services.

Stare, Fredrick J. "We're Flunking Food." In "Food & Fitness." Chicago: Blue Cross Assoc., 1973.

Stare, Fredrick J., Paul J. Cifrino and Jelia C. Witschi. "What Everyone Should Know About Nutrition." In "Food & Fitness." Chicago: Blue Cross Assoc., 1973.

"Food Is More Than Just Something To Eat." USDA, HEW, Grocery Manufacturers of America, Advertising Council, 1976.

U.S. Dept. of HEW. "The Cancer Quacks." Rptd. by American Cancer Society.

PUBLICATIONS AVAILABLE FROM THE
U.S. GOVERNMENT PRINTING OFFICE (Washington, D.C. 20402)

"Conserving the Nutritive Values In Food" (Home and Garden Bulletin No. 90).

Damon, G. Edward. "A Primer on Four Nutrients" (HEW Pub. No. (FDA) 75-2026).

Damon, G. Edward. "A Primer On Dietary Minerals" (Pub. No. (FDA) 75-2013).

"Family Fare: A Guide To Good Nutrition" (Home and Garden Bulletin No. 1).

Hecht, Annabel. "Hocus-Pocus As Applied to Arthritis" (HHS Pub. No. (FDA) 81-1080).

"How To Read A Food Label" (HEW Pub. No. (FDA) 80-1065).

Lehmann, Phyllis. "Food and Drug Interactions" (HEW Pub. No. (FDA) 80-3070).

"Metric Measures," HEW, 1976.

Morrison, Margaret. "A Consumer's Guide To Food Labels" (HEW Pub. No. (FDA) 77-2083).

Morrison, Margaret. "What About Vitamin C?" (Pub. No. (FDA) 75-2015).

"Myths of Vitamins," 1978.

"Nutrition and Your Health" (Home and Garden Bulletin No. 232).

"Nutrition Labels and U.S. RDA" (HEW Pub. No. (FDA) 76-2042).

Select Committee on Nutrition and Human Needs. "Dietary Goals For the United States." 2nd ed., 1977.

"Some Facts and Myths of Vitamins" (HEW Publication No. (FDA) 79-2117).

Stephenson, Marilyn. "The Confusing World of Health Foods" (HEW Pub. No. (FDA) 79-2108).

"Stubborn and Vexing, That's Acne" (HHS Pub. No. (FDA) 80-3107).

Taylor, Flora. "Aspirin: America's Favorite Drug" (HHS Pub. No. (FDA) 81-3115).

"Vitamin E—Miracle or Myth?" (DHEW Pub. No. (FDA) 76-2011).

Recommended Reading

Barrett, Stephen and Gilda Knight. *The Health Robbers.* Philadelphia: George F. Stickley, 1976.

Brody, Jane. *Jane Brody's Nutrition Book.* New York: W.W. Norton, 1981.

Consumer Guide. *The Vitamin Book.* New York: Simon and Schuster, 1979.

Food and Nutrition Board, National Academy of Sciences—National Research Council. *Recommended Dietary Allowances,* Ninth Edition. Washington, D.C.: National Academy of Sciences, 1980.

Hausman, Patricia. *Jack Sprat's Legacy: The Science and Politics of Fat & Cholesterol.* New York: Richard Marek Publishers, 1981.

Kreutler, Patricia A. *Nutrition In Perspective.* Englewood Cliffs, New Jersey: Prentice-Hall, Inc., 1980.

Labuza, Theodore P., ed. *The Nutrition Crisis.* St. Paul, Minnesota: West Publishing Co., 1975.

Labuza, Theodore P. and A. Elizabeth Sloan, eds. *Contemporary Nutrition Controversies.* St. Paul, Minnesota: West Publishing Co., 1979.

Levy, Joseph V. and Paul Bach-y-Rita. *Vitamins: Their Use And Abuse.* New York: Liveright, 1976.

Margolius, Sidney. *Health Foods: Facts and Fakes.* New York: Walker and Company, 1973.

McGill, Marion and Orrea Pye. *The No-Nonsense Guide to Food & Nutrition.* New York: Butterick Publishing, 1978.

About the Author

Virginia DeMoss is a graduate of the University of California and holds an M.A. degree in English from California State University, Long Beach. Ms. DeMoss was the Senior Editor for *Motorcyclist* and Managing Editor for *Cycle World*. She is presently a freelance writer/editor/photographer who contributes regularly to national publications; a number of her pieces on nutrition have appeared in *Runner's World* magazine.

In 1981 she was awarded the prestigious Maggie Award for magazine excellence.

TOTAL FITNESS BEGINS WITH THE RUNNER'S WORLD INSTRUCTIONAL SERIES.
Try It for 10 Days ... FREE

BEGIN YOUR TOTAL FITNESS PROGRAM TODAY
This one-of-a-kind instructional series is an innovative assembling of all you need to learn and enjoy on the way to total physical conditioning.

In your own home, you can master the ancient art of yoga ... eat better, feel stronger with a natural food diet ... massage stress and tightness from your weary muscles ... learn the fundamentals of weight lifting ... incorporate positive stretching into your daily workout ... and actualize total fitness with this complete instructional how-to series.

Every volume in the *Runner's World* Instructional Series is spiral-bound for easy application — designed to lie flat while you progress through our instructional programs. Each book is written by leading professionals and edited by the staff of *Runner's World*. You are assured of a format that is understandable and readable.

A 10-DAY FREE EXAMINATION OF EVERY VOLUME
Every volume in the *Runner's World* Instructional Series can expand your fitness horizons for a 10-day FREE examination. Here's how it works: If you decide to keep your introductory volume, we'll send you future volumes in the series approximately every other month — one volume at a time, always for a 10-day examination. You keep only the volumes you choose — there's no minimum number to buy — and you may cancel your subscription at any time simply by notifying us.

Beginning with the *Runner's World Yoga Book*, the series moves on to the *Indoor Exercise Book, Natural Foods Cookbook*, and more. Send for your introductory volume today.

EACH BOOK IN THE SERIES:
- Big 6½" × 9¼" format
- Spiral-bound for easy use
- Approximately 200 pages
- More than 150 photos and/or illustrations, all with easy, instructional, step-by-step formats
- Can be used with or without a partner
- Is specially priced at $9.95 ... a savings from publisher's retail price of $11.95
- Written by leading authorities and edited by the staff of *Runner's World*.

☐ YES, I would like to take advantage of a charter subscription to the *Runner's World* Instructional Book Series.

Please send my introductory volume for a 10-day free examination. If I decide to keep my introductory volume, I will pay $9.95 plus shipping and handling. I will then receive future volumes approximately every other month. Each volume is $9.95 plus shipping and handling and comes on the same 10-day free examination basis. There is no minimum number of books that I must buy, and I may cancel my subscription at any time simply by notifying you. If I do not choose to keep my initial selection I will return it within 10 days. My subscription for future volumes will be cancelled, and I will be under no further obligation.

Name_____

Address_____

City_____

State/Zip _____

Mail to:
Runner's World Instructional Book Series
1400 Stierlin Road
Mountain View, CA 94043

BUSINESS REPLY CARD

FIRST CLASS   PERMIT NO. 364   MTN. VIEW, CA

POSTAGE WILL BE PAID BY ADDRESSEE

Runner's World Instructional Book Series

1400 Stierlin Road
Mountain View, CA 94043